TAKING CHARGE

OF YOUR MEDICAL FATE

TAKING CHARGE

OF YOUR MEDICAL FATE

LAWRENCE C. HOROWITZ, M.D.

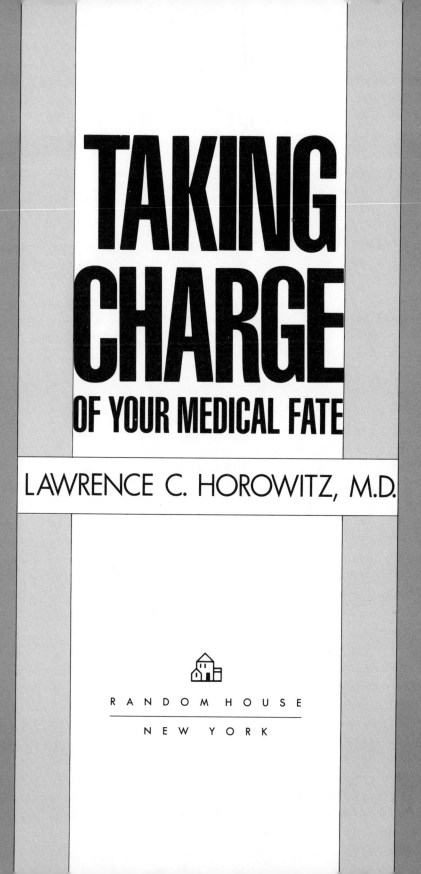

RANDOM HOUSE

NEW YORK

Grateful acknowledgment is made to the following for permission
to reprint previously published material:

Lexington Herald-Leader: A chart that appeared on page 85 of the September
1985 issue of the *Lexington Herald-Leader* (pp. 74–75).

The New York Times Company: A chart entitled "Above- or Below-Average U.S.
Mortality Rates" that apppeared in *The New York Times* on March 12, 1986.
Copyright © 1986 by The New York Times Company. Reprinted by permission.

Library of Congress Cataloging-in-Publication Data

Horowitz, Lawrence C.
Taking charge.

Includes index.
1. Medical care—United States. 2. Physician and
patient. 3. Consumer education. I. Title.
RA395.A3H65 1988 362.1'0973 88-2001
ISBN 0-394-56336-0

Manufactured in the United States of America
24689753
First Edition
BOOK DESIGN BY JOANNE METSCH

FOR LENORE

ACKNOWLEDGMENTS

This book is a synthesis of what many extraordinary people have taught me along the way. If the book has value, it is because their passionate commitment to trying to understand and improve the American health care system has value. I can't thank them all. And I can't thank them enough.

No one cares more about the quality of health care in America than Senator Edward Kennedy. His passion is genuine and personal, stemming from an extraordinary series of family medical problems that he knew would have bankrupted most other families. His professional commitment reaches back to the 1970s, when he first assumed responsibility for U.S. Senate oversight of most federal health care and biomedical research programs. He works harder on health care than on any other issue, and he has accomplished more to improve health care than anyone else in the Senate. I know because I was there—as a staff director of the health subcommittee and later as his overall chief of staff. The idea for this book grew out of a series of journeys across America, journeys that I took with Senator Kennedy to examine the American health care system. From urban to rural areas, from Indian reservations to migrant labor camps, from Orange County to Bedford Stuyvesant, the lessons were the same: Variability is at the center of the American way of health care—variability in quality of care, in access to care, in affordability of care. And many Americans—rich or poor, black, brown, yellow, or white—have something in common: They are unable to navigate through the system even when they have easy access to it.

No one better exemplifies what the phrase taking charge is about than Edward Bennett Williams. The title derives from my observations of his approach to life—to all aspects of it. Things don't happen to him without his taking charge, whether of the most difficult legal battles, political fights, or his own health care problems. He believes you must be in the arena, fighting to shape your own destiny. To put it another way, he accepts personal responsibility for what happens to him and around him. The acceptance and exercise of personal responsibility is at the heart of taking charge.

No training program has had a more profound influence on me than the Robert Wood Johnson Clinical Scholars Program at Stanford University. Located in the heart of the medical establishment, its purpose is to challenge the assumptions on which that establishment is based. Its director, Dr. Hal Holman, adheres to the thesis that things are seldom what they seem—and that with rigorous analysis, old conventions can be made to give way to new realities. Clinical scholars at Stanford learn both the limits of conventional wisdom and the unlimited potential of truly scientific human inquiry.

No single teacher has had more influence on me than Max Pepper, currently the chairman of the Department of Community Medicine at the St. Louis University School of Medicine. A professor during my medical school days at Yale University and a friend ever since, Max has shown me that a doctor's value is less in what he knows than in what he does with that knowledge. He was an activist at Yale, and he is an activist today. And while some might know more than Max Pepper, few have done more with what they knew.

No editor could have been more helpful or more understanding of what taking charge is all about than Charlotte Mayerson. She knew what I wanted to accomplish from the outset. She encouraged me; she challenged me; she sharpened the message. Charlotte knows firsthand about the variability of American medical care from her own and her family's illnesses. Yet in spite of the problems she has had, she believes in the basic message of this book: that by taking charge you can overcome the obstacles and live to see a brighter, healthier day ahead.

No agent could have done more to persuade a reluctant author of the value of his thesis than Sterling Lord. He believed in the message of this book from the first. He insisted on finding the right home—and the right editor—for it. And no book of this kind could have been written without meticulous research assistance. For me, that was provided by Dr. Michael Hensley in the early stages and then by Patricia Osborn, who put the text through a rigorous final check-up.

No author can be successful without the support and encouragement of his family. So to Essie and David, and also to Mirah, Jeremy, Michael, and Lauren Horowitz, I say a special thanks, for their unfailing faith in me to achieve what I set out to do.

Finally, and most important of all, no one who has written a book could have had a more important friend, both personally and professionally, than the woman to whom this book is dedicated. My wife is the best editor I have ever known, the most loyal and supportive person I have ever found, and the most loving. She knew what I wanted to say and has helped me to say it. She knows what I want to be, and she helps me to become it. Other men may be as lucky. But I doubt it.

CONTENTS

INTRODUCTION

"You're not better yet? You should see a doctor."

"You look terrible! You really should go to a doctor."

"I'm just not myself any more. I think I'd better see a doctor."

Common expressions. Common experiences. Shared by everyone—the old and the young, the rich and the poor.

All are based on a common assumption: When you're sick, when you need help, you can get it by going to a doctor.

And every day, acting on that assumption, patients in every city in America walk into their doctors' offices seeking help. And every day, in every city, the quality of the help they receive varies widely. Depending on how sick they are, on how serious their illnesses are, that variation can cost them prolonged suffering, extended illness, or even their lives.

For that assumption—when you're ill, you should go to a doctor—is wrong. And dangerous. If you're sick and need help, you need to select the right doctor, and by extension, the right hospital, the right laboratory, the right treatment. The purpose of this book is to convince you of that and to show you how to do it. The process is called taking charge.

We live in an increasingly standardized society. From the East Coast to the West Coast, we can walk into a Safeway supermarket confident that the white bread we purchase is of equal quality. A Ford purchased in Billings, Montana, will look just like the same model bought in Detroit. A General Electric refrigerator will keep the food as cold in a kitchen in San Francisco as in Buffalo. But human services are different. What people do cannot be standardized. We may try to set certain minimal standards for certain jobs, but people cannot be cloned.

Not all doctors are equally skillful. From state to state, from city to city, or hospital to hospital, doctors vary in how well they meet the needs of their patients. That variation can be enormous. Doctors vary in their diagnostic ability and in their technical ability to perform procedures. Some individuals are more familiar with new treatments and are better able to carry them out. How important these differences are to *you* depends on the nature of your problem.

Not as well known but equally significant is another kind of variation, the regional variation in the patterns of practice of groups of doctors. In some communities, most doctors are quick to recommend particular procedures or operations. In other communities, doctors would treat the same patients very differently, and the rate at which they perform the same operations or procedures is far lower. Both patterns of practice can't be right. But how is the patient to know which is wrong?

Most of the time, for most medical problems, the individual variations will not affect the outcome of your disease because most of your problems will turn out to be minor and self-limited. Whether you are treated optimally or not, chances are you will still get better. The more serious your illness, however, the more complicated it becomes, the more important proper treatment becomes, and the more harm can be done to you by the variability of medical care.

If you are seriously ill, if you have cancer or require open heart surgery or have any potentially life-threatening problem, *who* treats you and *where* you are treated can be more important to your survival than *what* you have. And those decisions—the who and the where—are entirely up to you. How carefully you make these choices may mean the difference between recovery and disability, between life and death.

There are people in America today who will lose their lives not because of their diseases but because they will choose one doctor's door to open rather than another's. It's not a question of malpractice, which certainly occurs but is relatively rare. It's more likely to be a question of the level of the doctor's knowledge, experience, and skill—qualities that vary in the delivery of all human services. It's just that in this area, those variations can have disastrous consequences.

Walking through a doctor's door without taking charge of the selection process is playing Russian roulette with your health. The quality of care in America may vary. The quality of *your care* doesn't have to. That's what this book is about.

The book is divided into three sections. The first makes the case for taking charge by showing you, with specific examples, why it is necessary. If you're not convinced of the need, you won't make the effort required to do it. The second section describes the obstacles to taking charge—obstacles inherent in the medical care system and in ourselves—that you will have to overcome if you are to be successful. The third section explains the process of taking charge. And it is a process, an approach to be followed, rather than a step-by-step recipe for each disease.

American medicine has more to offer than any other health care system in the world. But care is not offered equally by each doctor, nor is it needed equally by each patient. The challenge is to be sure that the doctor you visit has the capability to offer what you need. Whether your problem involves diagnosis or treatment, whether you need surgery or medication, whether you need primary or specialty care, the quality of your doctor will determine the quality of your care. That theme runs throughout the pages of this book. For that reason, because doctors are inseparable from all the different phases and forms of medical care, there is no separate section on physicians. All the sections are, at their core, about physicians.

I have seen taking charge save lives. During the ten years I spent in the United States Senate, first as staff director of the Senate Subcommittee on Health and Scientific Research and then as chief of staff for Senator Edward M. Kennedy, I encountered many senators and congressmen of both parties, and their constituents, who asked my help in solving difficult, often life-threatening medical problems. And all of them had the same questions: Where do I go? What do I do? How do I find the best doctor for the problem? None of them, no matter how famous or powerful, knew how to approach the problem alone. We helped them. What worked for them can work for you. That's the purpose of writing this book. What worked for them was taking charge.

SECTION ONE

WHY TAKING CHARGE IS CRITICAL TO YOUR HEALTH

HOSPITALS: HYSTERECTOMY AND CESAREAN SECTION

Hospitals. We think of them as the nerve centers of the American health care system. But the fact is that in America today, a hospital is a place that can save your life—or take it. At this moment, people are dying in hospitals who could be cured. People are being operated on who don't need to be. People are being hospitalized when there is no need for it.

We usually think of hospitals as places where most Americans are born, where serious illness is diagnosed, where we are repaired and restored, where emergencies are treated, and where many people inevitably die of their diseases. We think of hospitals as the high technology, high quality centers of the American health care system. And many of them are. But not all of them. In fact, very often the outcome of an illness depends more on the choice of doctor or hospital than on the disease itself.

How much does the quality of care vary from hospital to hospital? A lot! Consider this: In March of 1986, a minor action by the federal government created an enormous furor. The federal government published the death rates for Medicare patients in the nation's hospitals, and those rates varied enormously.

What follows is a copy of that list as it appeared in *The New York Times* on March 12, 1986. The list contains only those hospitals that had death rates either higher or lower than the national average, and compares those death rates with what should have been the case according to those national averages:

ABOVE- OR BELOW-AVERAGE U.S. MORTALITY RATES

Data tally the number of Medicare patients discharged from hospitals in 1984 and the percentage of those who died in the hospital. The hospitals listed are those with mortality rates that are higher or lower than average.

Hospitals not shown have mortality rates that are either in line with national averages or close enough to the averages so that the difference could easily be ascribed to chance.

The "forecast" percentage indicates how many patients would have been expected to die, according to national statistics partly adjusted for local conditions.

	Patients	Death Rate	Fore-cast
ALABAMA			
Lloyd Noland Hospital, Fairfield	2569	7.5	5.5
ARIZONA			
Maricopa Medical Center, Phoenix	2076	8.1	6.0
Community Hospital Medical Center, Phoenix	462	7.1	2.7
CALIFORNIA			
St. Helena Hospital & Health Center, Deer Park	2302	2.6	4.6
Mercy Hospital of Sacramento, Sacramento	5216	6.1	4.6
Grossmont District Hospital, La Mesa	6261	3.0	4.9
Oroville Hospital, Oroville	2137	6.7	4.6
Greater Bakersfield Memorial Hospital, Bakersfield	2305	8.1	4.9
Santa Clara Valley Medical Center, San Jose	1633	9.1	5.7

4

	Patients	Death Rate	Fore-cast
Samuel Merritt Hospital, Oakland	4660	6.0	4.2
Mercy Hospital & Medical Center, San Diego	7070	5.7	4.5
Brookside Hospital, San Pablo	2707	6.9	4.6
St. Francis Medical Center, Lynwood	4827	7.3	5.7
Palomar Memorial Hospital, Escondido	5096	7.3	5.3
Tri-City Hospital, Oceanside	5946	6.5	4.6
City of Hope National Medical Center, Duarte	1439	8.1	5.4
Long Beach Community Hospital, Long Beach	3439	6.9	5.1
Valley Medical Center of Fresno, Fresno	2401	9.5	7.2
Granada Hills Community Hospital, Granada Hills	2236	8.3	5.3
Pomona Valley Community Hospital, Pomona	4579	6.8	5.2
San Bernardino County Medical Center, San Bernardino	913	11.1	6.7
Redlands Community Hospital, Redlands	3339	7.7	6.1
Riverside General Hospital-University Medical Center, Riverside	1293	9.3	6.3
Mills Memorial Hospital, San Mateo	3992	5.1	7.0
Downey Community Hospital, Downey	2990	8.2	6.0
Eden Hospital, Castro Valley	2628	7.1	5.3
Mt. Diablo Hospital Medical Center, Concord	3843	6.3	4.9
Barlow Hospital, Los Angeles	131	18.3	4.0
CONNECTICUT			
New Milford Hospital, New Milford	1187	1.7	5.0
Hartford Hospital, Hartford	10051	7.2	5.9
Norwalk Hospital, Norwalk	4254	7.4	5.9

	Patients	Death Rate	Fore-cast
DISTRICT OF COLUMBIA			
Georgetown University Hospital, Washington	2219	1.9	5.4
Sibley Memorial Hospital, Washington	2777	2.9	4.8
FLORIDA			
Orlando Regional Medical Center, Orlando	7722	5.9	4.5
Doctors' Hospital, Coral Gables	3590	1.1	4.0
Bayfront Medical Center, St. Petersburg	4492	7.7	5.5
Holmes County Hospital, Bonifay	535	5.2	9.7
John F. Kennedy Memorial Hospital, Atlantis	6626	3.6	4.8
North Broward Medical Center, Pompano Beach	6742	6.2	4.6
Baptist Regional Health Services, Pensacola	4944	4.7	6.1
St. Luke's Hospital, Jacksonville	2606	2.6	4.9
Memorial Hospital, Ormond Beach	3772	5.3	6.9
Palm Beach Gardens Medical Center, Palm Beach Gardens	2737	7.5	5.1
Memorial Medical Center of Jacksonville, Jacksonville	4001	3.5	5.1
Humana Hospital Cypress, Pompano Beach	2880	5.6	3.7
GEORGIA			
Medical Center, Columbus	2901	7.0	5.1
Baldwin County Hospital, Milledgeville	1610	5.2	7.7
Clayton General Hospital	2955	3.1	4.9
HAWAII			
G. N. Wilcos Memorial Hospital & Health Center, Lihue	940	3.5	7.3

	Patients	Death Rate	Fore-cast
ILLINOIS			
University of Chicago Hospitals & Clinics, Chicago	3888	4.1	6.0
Northern Illinois Medical Center, McHenry	1795	4.3	6.7
Lutheran Hospital, Moline	2795	8.7	6.1
Cook County Hospital, Chicago	3343	1.9	5.5
Little Company of Mary Hospital, Evergreen Park	4967	6.8	5.4
St. Elizabeth's Hospital, Belleville	5847	6.6	5.2
Oak Forest Hospital of Cook County, Oak Forest	798	2.6	9.0
INDIANA			
Union Hospital, Terre Haute	5175	7.5	5.6
Methodist Hospital of Indiana, Indianapolis	8698	6.3	5.0
Broadway Methodist, Merrillville	2894	8.4	5.9
IOWA			
Muscatine General Hospital, Muscatine	1060	2.6	5.7
Boone County Hospital, Boone	1190	2.1	4.9
Mercy Hospital, Iowa City	2999	1.2	3.5
Mary Greeley Medical Center, Ames	2711	1.4	4.2
Mercy Hospital, Davenport	2592	2.2	4.9
Sartori Memorial Hospital, Cedar Falls	847	1.9	5.2
St. Luke's Methodist Hospital, Cedar Rapids	5025	1.5	3.8
University of Iowa Hospitals and Clinics, Iowa City	6199	1.7	3.7
St. Joseph Mercy Hospital, Mason City	3729	1.7	3.6
St. Francis Hospital, Waterloo	1922	1.2	4.3
Mercy Health Center, Dubuque	3537	1.9	4.8
Mercy Hospital, Cedar Rapids	3843	2.4	4.6

	Patients	Death Rate	Forecast
Iowa Methodist Medical Center, Des Moines	5969	1.8	4.3
Mercy Hospital Medical Center, Des Moines	6405	2.1	4.1
Broadlawns Medical Center, Des Moines	766	0.4	3.9
Des Moines General Hospital, Des Moines	2685	1.6	4.7
Davenport Osteopathic Hospital, Davenport	782	9.6	5.9
KANSAS			
University of Kansas Medical Center, Kansas City	3484	3.4	5.0
Greeley County Hospital, Tribune	91	20.9	10.0
St. Francis Reg. Medical Center, Wichita	8340	3.7	4.9
Holton City Hospital, Holton	177	12.4	5.4
KENTUCKY			
King's Daughter's Hospital, Ashland	3367	4.9	6.7
Methodist Hospital of Kentucky, Pikeville	2518	4.2	6.1
Owen County Memorial Hospital, Owenton	512	5.3	10.2
Western Baptist Hospital, Paducah	4272	6.6	5.2
LOUISIANA			
Huey P. Long Memorial Hospital, Pineville	524	9.4	5.3
Feliciana Medical Center, Clinton	656	4.1	8.1
Humana Hospital Springhill, Springhill	1262	7.1	4.2
Louisiana State University Hospital, Shreveport	2487	8.5	6.3
Humana Hospital Oakdale, Oakdale	908	6.2	3.0
Pendleton Memorial Methodist Hospital, New Orleans	2251	6.9	4.8

	Patients	Death Rate	Fore-cast
La Salle General Hospital, Jena	1339	2.8	6.0
River Parishes Medical Center, Laplace	745	10.2	4.6
MARYLAND			
Physicians' Memorial Hospital, La Plata	978	0.4	4.4
Maryland General Hospital, Baltimore	2328	1.8	5.0
Provident Hospital, Baltimore	1264	3.5	7.9
Lutheran Hospital of Maryland, Baltimore	1768	10.5	7.5
Greater Baltimore Medical Center, Baltimore	3690	2.7	4.2
MASSACHUSETTS			
Mount Auburn Hospital, Cambridge	3408	4.9	6.7
Union Hospital, Lynn	2352	2.5	5.9
Carney Hospital, Boston	4178	5.3	7.2
Hunt Memorial Hospital, Danvers	1208	2.4	5.6
Haverhill Mun-Hale Hospital, Haverhill	2020	9.1	6.4
Marlborough Hospital, Marlborough	1876	5.3	7.6
Charlton Memorial Hospital, Fall River	5174	6.4	8.2
Sancta Maria Hospital, Cambridge	1899	1.5	5.6
Baystate Medical Center, Springfield	8709	8.6	7.4
Glover Memorial Hospital, Needham	1320	0.5	4.6
Boston City Hospital, Boston	1538	0.2	5.9
Milton Hospital, Milton	2312	4.2	6.5
Faulkner Hospital, Boston	3417	5.1	7.7
Hahnemann Hospital, Boston	862	2.8	6.0
Falmouth Hospital, Falmouth	1764	5.7	7.9
Soldiers' Home in Holyoke, Holyoke	91	19.8	8.8
MICHIGAN			
Doctors Hospital, Detroit	720	14.2	7.3
Hurley Medical Center, Flint	3127	7.8	5.7

	Patients	Death Rate	Fore-cast
McLaren General Hospital, Flint	4586	5.4	6.8
Grand View Hospital, Ironwood	1020	3.9	7.7
Riverside Osteopathic Hospital, Trenton	1941	8.9	6.4
Oakland General Hospital Osteopathic, Madison Heights	2106	8.5	5.5
Chelsea Community Hospital, Chelsea	986	4.2	7.7
Southwest Detroit Hospital, Detroit	1397	9.8	6.1
MINNESOTA			
Regina Memorial Hospital, Hastings	569	4.6	8.4
St. Joseph's Hospital, St. Paul	2592	7.8	4.9
St. Paul-Ramsey Medical Center, St. Paul	3677	5.1	6.7
St. John's Hospital, St. Paul	2282	7.4	5.3
MISSISSIPPI			
Delta Medical Center, Greenville	1951	9.4	5.8
Greenwood Leflore Hospital, Greenwood	4229	1.5	2.9
Jeff Anderson Regional Medical Center, Meridian	3065	5.0	7.4
MISSOURI			
Lakeside Hospital, Kansas City	961	7.4	4.4
Jewish Hospital of St. Louis, St. Louis	7167	4.4	5.5
Bethesda General Hospital, St. Louis	1328	5.9	3.4
Pemiscot County Memorial Hospital, Hayti	1250	5.8	8.6
North Kansas City Memorial Hospital, North Kansas City	3493	6.5	4.6
St. Louis City Hospital, St. Louis	1171	12.3	9.4
MONTANA			
Missoula Community Hospital, Missoula	1232	1.7	4.3

	Patients	Death Rate	Fore-cast
NEBRASKA			
West Nebraska General Hospital, Scottsbluff	2978	5.9	3.8
Memorial Hospital, Aurora	513	9.9	3.3
NEVADA			
Humana Hospital Sunrise, Las Vegas	6768	6.0	4.9
Southern Nevada Memorial Hospital, Las Vegas	2650	7.8	5.6
Adelson Hospice, Las Vegas	169	87.6	22.5
NEW JERSEY			
Newark Beth Israel Medical Center, Newark	4146	8.0	6.3
Cooper Hospital-University Medical Center, Camden	3851	10.1	6.3
Christ Hospital, Jersey City	3486	9.3	7.4
St. Joseph's Hospital & Medical Center, Paterson	5536	9.2	7.1
Deborah Heart and Lung Center, Browns Mills	1702	3.8	5.9
Millville Hospital, Millville	1697	8.7	5.7
Community Memorial Hospital, Toms River	7797	9.0	7.8
St. Francis Hospital, Jersey City	2637	9.0	7.2
Zurbrugg Memorial Hospital, Willingboro	2365	8.1	5.9
Muhlenberg Hospital, Plainfield	3996	8.0	6.5
St. Peter's Medical Center, New Brunswick	4199	8.4	7.0
Jersey Shore Medical Center, Neptune	5720	9.7	8.1
Jersey City Medical Center, Jersey City	1782	11.3	8.1
Monmouth Medical Center, Long Branch	4668	9.5	6.8

	Patients	Death Rate	Fore-cast
Kennedy Memorial Hospitals University Medical Center, Stratford	5847	8.9	6.8
NEW YORK			
Peninsula Hospital Center, Far Rockaway	3818	12.5	9.7
Bronx-Lebanon Hospital Center, Bronx	2681	6.5	8.4
Presbyterian Hospital in New York, New York	9646	6.4	7.4
Nassau County Medical Center, East Meadow	3825	14.7	9.7
St. Jerome Hospital, Batavia	1608	6.7	9.0
Southside Hospital, Bay Shore	4383	10.7	8.4
Roosevelt Hospital, New York	4104	5.9	8.4
St. Peter's Hospital, Albany	4916	10.9	8.9
Montefiore Medical Center, Bronx	13227	6.2	7.1
Lincoln Medical Mental Health Center, Bronx	1743	13.0	10.0
New York Eye and Ear Infirmary, New York	5689	0.0	2.1
North Shore University Hospital, Manhasset	6084	10.2	8.7
Yonkers General Hospital, Yonkers	2884	9.2	7.4
Bronx Municipal Hospital Center, Bronx	4256	12.2	7.9
City Hospital Center at Elmhurst, Flushing	3451	16.7	14.1
St. Joseph's Hospital Health Center, Syracuse	5499	10.3	8.8
Little Falls Hospital, Little Falls	1563	8.6	6.2
Ellis Hospital, Schenectady	5154	8.1	6.6
House of the Good Samaritan, Watertown	2585	9.1	6.9
Beth Israel Medical Center, New York	6230	2.5	6.2

	Patients	Death Rate	Fore-cast
Community Hospital at Glen Cove, Glen Cove	3145	10.1	8.0
New Rochelle Hospital Medical Center, New Rochelle	4318	9.2	7.5
Glens Falls Hospital, Glens Falls	5970	5.7	7.0
Flushing Hospital and Medical Center, Flushing	4170	12.4	9.5
Maimonides Medical Center, Brooklyn	7213	9.2	7.8
Kings County Hospital Center, Brooklyn	2285	14.5	10.5
New York University Medical Center, New York	6755	4.4	6.5
Queens Hospital Center, Jamaica	2741	12.7	10.2
Harlem Hospital Center, New York	2479	15.0	9.9
Champlain Valley Physicians Hospital Medical Center, Plattsburgh	4662	6.0	7.9
Osteopathic Hospital, Flushing	2961	13.9	10.1
Medical Arts Center Hospital, New York	462	2.6	8.2
Strong Memorial Hospital Rochester University, Rochester	5379	6.0	7.5
Good Samaritan Hospital, West Islip	4759	10.6	9.2
Julia L. Butterfield Memorial Hospital, Cold Spring	512	4.9	9.2
St. Vincent's Hospital & Medical Center, New York	5760	8.9	7.3
Lake Shore Hospital, Irving	697	10.8	6.8
Parsons Hospital, Flushing	1549	13.8	9.0
Prospect Hospital, Bronx	851	1.8	5.0
Tompkins Community Hospital, Ithaca	2284	3.7	7.1
Smithtown General Hospital, Smithtown	2639	10.7	8.3
Pelham Bay General Hospital, Bronx	2043	10.6	8.1
Roswell Park Memorial Institute, Buffalo	2176	5.1	6.9

	Patients	Death Rate	Fore-cast
Hospital for Joint Diseases, New York	1352	0.0	2.6
Joint Diseases North General Hospital, New York	869	3.5	7.0
United Health Services, Johnson City	8995	5.5	6.8
St. Johns Episcopal Hospital, Garden City	5692	9.0	7.7
Interfaith Medical Center, Brooklyn	2876	12.7	8.5
NORTH CAROLINA			
Hoots Memorial Hospital, Yadkinville	574	3.1	7.7
Scotland Memorial Hospital, Laurinburg	1212	4.5	7.1
Forsyth Memorial Hospital, Winston-Salem	8988	7.5	6.3
Morehead Memorial Hospital, Eden	1264	2.1	5.3
Frye Regional Medical Center, Hickory	2036	2.0	5.1
Granville Hospital, Oxford	617	10.2	6.3
Huntersville Hospital, Huntersville	125	19.2	8.3
OHIO			
Mercy Hospital of Hamilton, Hamilton	3804	3.5	5.4
Mercy Medical Center, Springfield	3085	4.8	6.6
Blanchard Valley Hospital, Findlay	2759	4.3	6.4
Fostoria City Hospital, Fostoria	929	4.1	7.2
City Hospital, Bellaire	1326	3.9	6.5
Bethesda North Hospital, Cincinnati	8188	7.3	6.1
OKLAHOMA			
Grand Valley Hospital, Pryor	1240	7.3	4.2
South Community Hospital, Oklahoma City	4535	5.8	4.2

	Patients	Death Rate	Fore-cast
OREGON			
Sacred Heart General Hospital, Eugene	5809	1.4	4.0
PENNSYLVANIA			
Geisinger Medical Center, Danville	6911	1.5	3.8
North Penn Hospital, Lansdale	1999	3.0	5.1
Evangelical Community Hospital, Lewisburg	2399	3.0	5.3
St. Agnes Medical Center, Philadelphia	2487	7.6	5.5
Chestnut Hill Hospital, Philadelphia	3221	4.3	6.3
Hahnemann University Hospital, Philadelphia	4662	5.8	4.5
Franklin Regional Medical Center, Franklin	4026	3.6	5.0
Lancaster General Hospital, Lancaster	7034	4.6	6.0
Hospital of the University of Pennsylvania, Philadelphia	5447	3.4	5.1
Suburban General Hospital, Norristown	1733	1.7	4.6
Mercy Catholic Medical Center, Darby	5935	5.2	6.4
Haverford Community Hospital, Havertown	1258	3.5	6.7
Abington Memorial Hospital, Abington	6645	5.2	6.4
Hanover General Hospital, Hanover	2178	3.7	6.6
Episcopal Hospital, Philadelphia	2398	3.2	5.3
Milton S. Hershey Medical Center, Hershey	3300	4.3	6.1
St. Mary Hospital, Langhorne	2127	3.2	6.0
RHODE ISLAND			
Westerly Hospital, Westerly	1976	5.5	7.9

	Patients	Death Rate	Fore-cast
SOUTH CAROLINA			
Medical University Hospital, Charleston	2649	2.4	4.2
North Trident Regional Hospital, Charleston	2901	2.6	5.2
TENNESSEE			
Methodist-Hospital Central Unit, Memphis	14615	5.8	4.9
Maury County Hospital, Columbia	3757	2.6	4.6
Regional Medical Center at Memphis, Memphis	1578	11.1	8.2
TEXAS			
Dallas County Hospital District, Dallas	3559	7.7	5.6
R. E. Thomason General Hospital, El Paso	720	10.0	6.4
St. Paul Hospital, Dallas	4652	2.4	4.8
Southeast Baptist Hospital, San Antonio	12123	5.9	5.0
Hermann Hospital, Houston	4647	6.5	4.8
St. Mary Hospital, Port Arthur	3217	9.0	4.5
Mesquite Physicians Hospital, Mesquite	996	9.7	6.3
Memorial Hospital, Lufkin	2970	0.2	3.4
Hopkins County Memorial Hospital, Sulphur Springs	1787	7.8	5.2
Harris County Hospital District, Houston	1376	11.2	8.2
Rosewood General Hospital, Houston	1445	4.1	7.8
Southwest Osteopathic Hospital, Amarillo	566	10.1	5.8
Richardson Medical Center, Richardson	969	2.7	6.2
Spring Branch Memorial Hospital, Houston	1287	0.6	3.3

	Patients	Death Rate	Fore-cast
Valley Community Hospital, Brownsville	854	0.8	4.0
VIRGINIA			
University of Virginia Hospital & Children Rehabilitation, Charlottesville	5368	3.3	4.9
St. Luke's Hospital, Richmond	2404	6.3	4.4
King's Daughters' Hospital, Staunton	2396	7.6	5.4
Riverside Hospital, Newport News	4868	7.0	5.3
Grundy Hospital, Grundy	923	2.4	5.8
WASHINGTON			
Swedish Hospital Medical Center, Seattle	8778	5.3	4.0
Shorewood Osteopathic Hospital, Seattle	266	10.2	4.4
WEST VIRGINIA			
Bluefield Community Hospital, Bluefield	3877	0.9	3.1
WISCONSIN			
St. Mary's Hospital, Milwaukee	2965	9.0	6.1
Mount Sinai Medical Center, Milwaukee	3778	7.3	5.3
St. Joseph's Hospital, Milwaukee	5605	8.8	7.3
WYOMING			
Memorial Hospital of Natrona County, Casper	1891	7.0	4.5

Nothing like this had ever been published in America before, and predictably, the medical and hospital associations were outraged. There were explanations for the figures, they said. And in part they were right. There were explanations—for some. Federal officials conceded that perhaps as many as half the variations could be explained. But after all the explanations, after all the arguments, after all the limitations for the statistics were pointed out, one overriding fact remained: There is real variability in the quality of health care from hospital to hospital in America, and this variability is reflected in the rate at which people die while under care.

Need more evidence? There's a lot more. At the same time that the overall death rates were released, the federal government released other data to show how elderly people with nine common diseases fared at the nation's hospitals. How they fared, whether they recovered or died from diseases such as pneumonia or operations such as bypass surgery, varied from hospital to hospital. In fact, the figures show that for a comparable disease, a patient's chance of dying in some of these hospitals is several times greater than in others. The disease can be the same. The person's condition can be the same. But the outcome can be as different as life and death, depending on where you go.

How do we Americans make the potentially fateful choice of which hospital to go to? Often the doctor makes it for us. We go where he puts us,* usually on faith and without an independent assessment on our part. Often we go because of geographic proximity to where we live. Sometimes there is no choice. In emergencies we go where we are taken or to the closest possible place. But when there is the potential for choice, effectively taking charge requires that we be active participants in the process. Our interests and our doctor's may not totally coincide. He has to practice where he has staff privileges; we have the right to go where we want, where we have the best chance to achieve the right result.

---

*Although the number of women physicians is growing, men still substantially outnumber women in this profession. For that reaso, the masculine pronouns shall be used to refer to both male and female physicians.

The decision as to where to go can be a life-or-death one; the decision as to whether or not to go into a hospital can be a very expensive one. And how that decision gets made varies widely as well. As many as 40 percent of hospital admissions may be unnecessary. That is, the treatment could have been properly given outside the hospital, according to a recent study by the Rand Corporation. Whether or not the admission is necessary depends on your doctor and, often, on your insurance. But the decision to hospitalize should not be taken lightly, and taking charge requires full participation in it.

If hospitals are the crown jewels of the American health care system, surgeons are its royal family. American surgeons are the most talented in the world, and at its best, surgery in America can be nothing short of miraculous. It can also be life-threatening. What one surgeon does well, another does poorly. *Your* challenge is to find the right one for your operation. It's not just the surgeon's technical skill that is at issue here; it is his judgment about when to operate and when not to. Among doctors, it is well known that some surgeons are "quick to cut" and others "cut only as a last resort." Those reputations are independent of the medical conditions of the patients.

It is less well known that in some locations almost all the surgeons are "quicker to cut" than in other areas. Consider this: John Wennberg and Alan Gittelsohn compared two cities in Maine, less than twenty miles from each other, and found an astounding difference in the rate at which hysterectomies were performed—even though general health conditions in the two cities were comparable.[1] A woman living in city A, for example, would have been almost three times more likely to have her uterus removed before she was seventy-five years old than a woman living in city B. Imagine that you are female, living in city A. The hysterectomy rate there is so high that if it continued, you would have a 70 percent chance of having your uterus removed by the time you were seventy-five years old. In city B, your chances of losing your uterus would be 25 p .cent.

What can account for this difference? Wennberg and Gittelsohn found it was not economic conditions; they were similar. The difference was not in the number of physicians or in the supply of hospital beds. It wasn't even a difference in the health status of the patients, or in the coverage of their health insurance plans. So what could account for such an enormous difference in hysterectomy rates? According to the authors, "The most important factor in determining the rate of hysterectomy seems to be the style of medical practice of the physicians in the two cities. In one city surgeons *appear to be enthusiastic about hysterectomy; in the other they appear to be skeptical of its value* [emphasis added]."

How would you feel playing this kind of roulette, where your place of birth would have more impact on whether you undergo a hysterectomy than your medical condition? The fact is that the rates in both cities could reflect poor quality care—too low in one, too high in the other. But the main point is the enormous variation, and how little of that variation is based on scientific fact, and therefore how important it is to take charge, to understand the options and choose for yourself. The doctors in both these cities clearly believe their approach to be best. But they can't both be right. They can, in fact, both be wrong. The last section of this book will show you how to determine what the best scientific evidence is so that you can make the most informed decision for your individual medical problem.

The Wennberg-Gittelsohn study looked at other forms of surgery as well. In fact, it looked at surgical rates in 193 small areas within a six-state region of New England. Wennberg and Gittelsohn found as much as a fourfold variation in prostatectomy rates and a sixfold variation in tonsillectomy rates. Your chances of losing your tonsils, or your prostate, or your gall bladder vary greatly from area to area, *independent* of your medical conditions. Why? "Style of medical practice" of local physicians seems to be the reason. "Style" is not science. It is often based more on custom and intuition than on scientific evidence. Wennberg and Gittelsohn discovered that practice areas are marked with "surgical signatures" that remain constant over the years. That is, just as Detroit is an "automobile" town and Washington, D.C., is a "government" town, some medical areas are "hysterectomy" towns and some are "gall bladder" towns. In three different areas of Maine, for example, the overall rate of surgery was almost the same, but in each of the three areas, the most common procedure was different! In fact, what was commonest in one area was least common in the other. Why? "Style of practice."

The consequences of these variations can be more profound than the potential of needlessly losing a body part. A consequence might also be premature death—because surgery, any surgery, has risks. For many surgical procedures, that risk includes the development of complications leading to death. Unnecessary surgery leads to unnecessary deaths.

The Wennberg-Gittelsohn study clearly shows the enormous impact that surgical rates can have on deaths. For example, if the highest surgical rate for prostatectomy in Maine were applied nationwide, then 6,800 men undergoing that procedure in 1975 would have died of surgical complications. On the other hand, if the lowest rate of prostatectomy found in Maine were applied to the whole country, only 1,900 men would have died. That difference—five thousand deaths that could have been avoided—

would be based on style of practice. Hypothetical example? Yes. But variability in surgical rates most certainly exists—from town to town, from state to state, from country to country. And although the variations are not dependent on medical condition, or on scientific indications for surgery, they have profound impact on the health and well-being and the very lives of all of us.

These variations are not a unique characteristic of American medicine; they exist wherever medicine is practiced. For example, Wennberg, John Bunker, and Benjamin Barnes compared surgical rates for seven very common procedures in Canada, the United Kingdom, and in different U.S. geographic areas. Hysterectomy rates varied sixfold from one place to another, tonsillectomy rates varied sixfold, gall bladder surgery varied ninefold, prostatectomy varied eightfold, hemorrhoidectomy varied seven and a halffold. Overall for the seven procedures, there was a fivefold variation between the highest rate area and the lowest. Rates varied within countries and between them. Rates were lowest in the United Kingdom, highest in Canada.[2]

What is the significance? The more surgery that is performed, the more deaths occur as complications. If the surgery is necessary, the risks are justified. If the surgery is not necessary, the deaths are needless. The difference between the high rates and low rates, if extrapolated nationally, is thousands and thousands of deaths a year.

And, to repeat, where you live, the "style of practice" in your area, determines your risk, often independent of your medical condition.

Why does this happen? Isn't there a right and wrong way to do things? The answer has to do with the nature of the practice of medicine, with the old dichotomy—is it an art or a science? The truth is, medicine is closer to an art that is based on science.

And the effort to make it more scientific—to assess the outcomes of common medical practices in order to know what is correct and what isn't—goes on all the time. But as Wennberg, Bunker, and Barnes state in their paper:

> Medical innovations have not generally been subjected to rigorous evaluation prior to their widespread use by the medical community. As a result, a good deal of uncertainty and disagreement exists among physicians concerning the value of many common practices in all fields of medicine—uncertainty and disagreement which is in turn reflected in the large variations in therapeutic practices among physicians.

Each year, the science of medicine advances, and there is greater understanding of what works and what doesn't. There is a lag, however, between the development of a new understanding and the change of medical practice to reflect it. "Styles of practice" become ingrained and hard to change. Taking charge will help you understand what is known and what is not, and what your options are. You should never be a captive of the style of practice in your area. You may choose to be treated in that area, but you should do so only after knowing how others approach the same problem—what your options are. As the Wennberg study concludes:

> The limits on informed decision-making in medical markets are more severe than is generally realized. . . . Informed decision making is particularly problematic when an intervention is undertaken to improve in some uncertain way the quality of life, when the trade-off involves an increased risk of immediate death or iatrogenic complication, and when

there is little or no expected increase in life-expectancy. When decisions are made, whose values are being expressed, the patient's or the physician's? The geographic variations in exposure rates are consistent with the thesis that medical care choices are highly dependent on the preferences of physicians. When professional disagreement is strong, and patients delegate decision-making to physicians, the probability of exposure to specific intervention will often depend on the style of practice of the physician or clinic selected for care rather than the nature and severity of the illness.

It is a hard concept to accept that the treatment you receive, or your decision to have surgery, or even, in some cases, your chance of dying prematurely in a hospital depends more on which doctor's door you walk through than on the illness inside your body. There is no more compelling justification for the need for taking charge. If a medical decision is to be made on the basis of style of practice rather than a scientific standard, and if the different options have similar chances for success, then your judgment is as good, as valid, as your doctor's. If the decision is to be based on science rather than style, then you also have an obligation to be a partner in the decision-making process. All physicians want to do right by their patients. The problem is that many times there are different views of what's right. And although a surgeon can change his view over time, and even change his approach to particular diseases as the medical evidence changes, you, as the patient undergoing surgery, never get a second chance. Taking charge is about maximizing the chances for success the first time.

Not only does the rate at which surgical procedures are performed vary greatly from area to area, but these rates can also change significantly over time in the same area. Where certain operations were once common, they might now be performed far less frequently. What is thought to be the right approach today may be considered wrong tomorrow. The state of medical practice is dynamic, and sometimes the treatments our children receive are very different from the ones we received for the same problems. In few types of surgical practice are the differences over time and the differences between areas so pronounced as with hysterectomies. Earlier we showed that in two similar cities in Maine, twenty miles apart, the chances of a woman reaching age seventy-five with her uterus intact varied between 25 and 70 percent. Obviously, when you talk about the overall hysterectomy rate in the state of Maine, you miss these sharp area variations. Even so, the aggregate rates still vary from state to state and region to region.

HYSTERECTOMY

By the end of the seventies, surgical removal of the uterus had become the commonest major surgical procedure performed on a daily basis in the U.S. The rapid rise to the top occurred between 1970 and 1975, when the rate rose by 33 percent, according to a study by Alexander Walker and Hershel Jick. Not only did the numbers rise, but they rose for all age groups under sixty-five years. And once again, where you lived had an enormous impact on whether or not you had this operation. If you were female and under thirty-five years of age in 1975, your chances of losing your uterus that year were three times higher if you lived in the South than in the Northeast. But even in the Northeast, the number of hysterectomies rose from 115,000 in 1970 to 136,000 in 1975. In the North Central states, the rate was 168,000 in 1970 and 199,000 in 1975. In the West, the rate went up from 122,000 in 1970 to 143,000 in 1975. In the South, 214,000 hysterectomies were performed in 1970; 245,000 in 1971; 260,000 in 1972, and 303,000 in 1975.[3]

Why are there such variations over time and between areas? The answer lies in the reasons for which hysterectomies are performed: cancer, benign fibroid tumors, pelvic relaxation, uterine bleeding, diseases of the ovaries and fallopian tubes. And hysterectomies are also performed for prophylaxis, on the theory that where there's no uterus, there will be no cancer, or no uterus, no more children.

For some of these indications, all doctors would agree that hysterectomies are necessary. But for the majority, opinion varies widely and so does the rate of surgery. As Thomas Koepsell and his colleagues discovered when they studied hysterectomy rates in Seattle and Tacoma, "The controversy over appropriate indications and the preponderance of benign uterine disease for which non-surgical treatment alternatives are often available have complicated both the physician's decision as to whether to recommend hysterectomy and the patient's decision as to whether to accept it. Thus, performance of a hysterectomy is often discretionary on medical grounds, and an opportunity is created for non-biological factors, such as the nature and extent of a woman's insurance coverage, to play a major role."[4]

Thus on one end of the spectrum—hysterectomy for cancer—there is full medical unanimity. On the other end—hysterectomy as prophylaxis against conditions that may never occur—there is vigorous disagreement. In the middle are many conditions for which alternatives to surgery exist.

Hysterectomy as prophylaxis? Hysterectomy as a convenience? Hard to believe? But it is happening. The decision to have this operation for these reasons is not a medical one; it has to do with life-style. It should not be your doctor's decision. It should be yours. Sometimes it is appropriate for a given person in a given situation, but it can never be appropriate if the decision to go ahead results from physician pressure. That pressure may reflect a physician's personal judgment about your personal life-style, or it may reflect the coverage of your insurance policy.

As with all truly elective surgery, and major surgery at that, it is your choice. You are in the best position to make it, and you are *more capable* of making it in your own best interests than is your doctor.

Hysterectomy for benign conditions where medical alternatives exist? The right decision for some, the wrong one for others, but here again, it is your decision. You must understand the medical options and medical consequences. You can and should give serious consideration to your doctor's medical judgment. But your decision should not be determined for you by the "style of practice" in the place where you live. It should be determined by an objective assessment of what's right for you. Taking charge requires that you take control of the decision-making process.

Major surgery is never without risk. Hysterectomy risks are not just physical; they can be psychological and emotional as well. Such side effects can be very difficult to treat. And they may be unnecessary. Many of the uteri examined in the pathology laboratory after they have been removed do in fact look completely normal, with no physical abnormalities whatsoever. Dr. Nancy Lee and her colleagues have studied more than 1,800 women who had undergone hysterectomy. More than half (52 percent) of these women underwent surgery because of a diagnosis that was medically precise enough that it could theoretically have been confirmed by laboratory study of the uterus. Of all these potentially confirmable diagnoses, a full 8 percent of the uteri were found after surgery to be completely normal on pathologic examination.[5]

For the 48 percent of women who had hysterectomies for diagnoses that could not be expected to be confirmed by laboratory study—general diagnoses such as menstrual bleeding disorders, pelvic pain, or pelvic relaxation—a full 38 percent of these uteri were found after surgery to be completely normal in every respect on pathologic examination. In these cases, as with the 8 percent in the first group, one must wonder what the cause of the symptoms was—and whether the removal of a perfectly normal uterus was the right solution.

To put it another way, the more medically precise the diagnosis, the more likely a diseased uterus will be removed. The more general the diagnosis, pelvic pain for example, the more likely a perfectly healthy uterus will be removed. And in those cases, not included in the Lee study, where hysterectomy is performed prophylactically, by definition the uterus removed will have no abnormalities.

Once again this problem is not unique to America. According to a report in 1984 in the *British Journal of Obstetrics and Gynecology*, nearly half the patients who underwent an abdominal hysterectomy in one district hospital in Great Britain in 1980 had perfectly normal, healthy uteri upon pathologic examination. The authors concluded:

> There is a need for more understanding of the causes of dysfunctional uterine haemorrhage and enigmatic pelvic pain so that less radical therapy can be developed.

The authors expressed concern about the increasing incidence of hysterectomy in their areas, particularly "in view of the reported adverse long-term psychiatric and cardiovascular effects of hysterectomy."[6]

What does all this mean? It means *beware*. It means the medical profession is unsettled and divided over when to perform a hysterectomy. It means the conventional wisdom of today may change tomorrow. It means that "style of practice" rather than objective scientific information may be responsible for your physician's recommendation.

In the past, radical mutilating surgery for breast cancer was the vogue. In most areas, with the best of intentions, and with the belief in its scientific merit, doctors unnecessarily performed this deforming surgery. Today those same doctors, and their successors, *don't*, and they shake their heads about what used to be.

Today hysterectomies are on the rise and are done for many reasons, some scientific and medically necessary and some not. Tomorrow your doctor may view things very differently and shake his head about what used to be. It is a reflection of the nature of medical practice. But it is very hard to accept that what our doctor currently believes and recommends with the best of intentions may in fact be wrong, and that we may suffer the consequences.

In medicine, there are few certainties. There are more questions than answers. There are few truths. And everything is changing. Most of the time, the best we can hope for is the best judgment based on the best available facts and the particular circumstances. And the best judgment is seldom obtained by delegating the responsibility for it to the physician alone. The best judgment, and thus the best chance for success, depends on your taking charge.

CESAREAN SECTION

Cesarean section has become almost as controversial as hysterectomy, partly because the American way of birth has been changing so dramatically. Fifty years ago the majority of Americans were born at home, but by 1970, 99.4 percent of all births took place in a hospital.[7] Even the recent revival of interest in home delivery has had a negligible impact on that trend. Initially most hospital births were delivered vaginally. In the last fifteen years, however, abdominal surgery—cesarean section—has increased more than threefold. The increases have been extraordinary, from 4.5 percent of all births in 1965 to 17.9 percent for all ages in 1981. More alarming is that the rate for women over thirty-five went from 7.9 percent to 24.4 percent, a threefold increase to almost one in four births![8]

In 1986, 906,000 women in the country had C-sections, accounting for 24 percent of all births. Almost one of every four Americans is now born in surgery, by a C-section. But behind these staggering numbers are the same questions, the same need for taking charge. Here too, where you live and the kind of hospital you go to will influence the decision to have a C-section —and ultimately, the outcome of the surgery as well.

What is not clear is whether these huge numbers reflect good medical practice, and increasingly, voices are being raised against the trend. According to several recent studies, too many C-sections are being performed and for the wrong reasons, causing unnecessary complications to the mother and child.

Why? Clearly obstetricians have no intention of putting their

1984 C-SECTION RATE BY REGION AND TYPE OF HOSPITAL (PERCENT)

Area	Total	Proprietary Hospitals	Government Hospitals	Nonprofit Hospitals
U.S.	17.9	22.0	15.4	18.5
Northeast	20.0	25.5	14.9	20.4
North Central	15.9	30.4	14.5	15.9
South	18.8	18.9	15.8	20.4
West	17.1	22.5	15.5	17.4

patients at unnecessary risk. The answer is that obstetricians do not believe they are, and won't believe it until the current patterns of practice have lasted long enough and been studied extensively enough that definitive indications for C-sections can be recommended and agreed to. Then the pendulum will undoubtedly swing back somewhat. But it is hard to say when that will happen, and it is of little value to those of you who face childbirth decisions now.

The increase in C-sections corresponds to the advances in medical technology and the improvement in surgical and postsurgical care. With new technology, we can detect fetal problems that were undetectable fifteen years ago. We can safely deliver by C-section babies who would have died otherwise. The surgery today is far safer, the complications far fewer than they were. There are risks, though they are far more acceptable today than they used to be. To put it simply, the proper goal of C-sections is to improve the chances of babies at risk, and that goal has been achieved.

But as with everything in medicine, there is another side to the coin. Just because C-sections are much safer than they used to be doesn't mean they are safe enough to be considered routinely as an elective option for most births. After all, C-sections are surgical procedures, and the chance of a woman's dying during a C-section is two to four times greater than during a vaginal delivery. The procedure carries risks, for both the mother and the baby. The decision to have a C-section should always be a risk-versus-benefit decision geared to each individual case. When the risks incurred outweigh the likely benefits, then any procedure is out of place. So an appropriate procedure to improve the chances of a baby at risk can be inappropriate if the motivation is simply the convenience of the mother or doctor.

Although the United States leads the industrialized world in its C-section rate—50 to 200 percent higher than in most other countries—rates are rising everywhere and so is concern about them. In 1987, Dr. Marion Hall of the Aberdeen Maternity Hospital in the United Kingdom wrote in the *British Medical Journal* that C-sections should not be performed once labor has begun without a major medical indication. The reason? Studies in England and Wales have shown that "in women whose pregnancies reach the stage of delivery, both direct and indirect death rates are about ten times higher when delivery is by caesarean section rather than vaginal. Some deaths are, of course, caused by the condition that was indicated for the operation, but at least half are caused *by the operation itself* [emphasis added]."9

Unquestionably the so-called "emergency" C-sections—those undertaken after labor has begun—have a higher mortality and morbidity rate than elective procedures for the mother. But the fetus must also be considered, and there is a price to be paid for scheduling elective C-sections in order to avoid those that may become necessary after labor has begun. As Hall points out:

Elective caesarean section is relatively safer . . . for the mother but not for the fetus, with risks to respiratory function and intellectual development. To the immediate hazards of any caesarean section must be added the enhanced risk in a subsequent pregnancy of requiring another operative delivery or of developing placenta praevia. Fertility is also reduced.

In the United States, the maternal death rate after cesarean sections in the state of Georgia was 59.3 deaths per 100,000 C-sections, according to a study headed by George L. Rubin.[10] Complication rates are even higher. Thorkild Neilsen and his colleagues reported a complication rate of 24.2 percent in emergency C-sections and 4.7 percent in elective C-sections.[11] And O. H. Jones reported similar, even higher complication rates at Charlotte Memorial Hospital, a large southern metropolitan hospital. These included uncontrollable bleeding requiring hysterectomy, postoperative bleeding, vaginal fistula, ureteral fistula and obstruction, bladder perforations, lacerated intestines, pelvic abscess, hematoma, thrombophlebitis, wound infection, and morbidity.[12]

What does this mean? It means that if you are pregnant, you ought to participate actively in the decision whether to have a C-section. It means that the procedure will often be recommended as necessary or desirable when it isn't. It means that, if you are not taking charge, you may undergo needless surgery with needless risk to yourself and your child.

C-sections have saved countless lives. They will save countless more. All would agree to that. But increasingly, there is agreement that too many are being done for too little justification. It is even true that as time goes on, we are finding that reasons for which C-sections were once thought to be absolutely necessary and unequivocally beneficial are now open to question. One such reason is when the baby is lying feet down, in what is called the frank breech position. Twenty years ago these babies were delivered vaginally most of the time. By 1980, however, they were delivered by C-section most of the time. According to Dr. Sidney Bottoms and his colleagues, writing in *The New England Journal of Medicine* in 1980, "this dramatic change in management is understandable since the benefit of selective abdominal delivery for the fetus in breech presentation is perhaps easier to document than benefit from cesarean birth for any other frequent indication."[13] Case closed? No. Writing in *The American Journal of Obstetrics and Gynecology* in the same year, Dr. Joseph Collea reached very different conclusions. After studying the outcomes of C-section and vaginal deliveries for 208 breech cases, he and his colleagues found a "striking and concerning" incidence of maternal morbidity in the C-section deliveries compared with the vaginal deliveries: "Despite modern operative techniques and systemic antibiotic regimens, women undergoing cesarean section in our institution experience intraoperative complications, blood loss, and infectious morbidity at a rate much higher than those associated with vaginal delivery. Maternal risks of morbidity multiply when one considers the potential anesthetic and operative complications encountered in subsequent abdominal deliveries." The outcomes of all 208 pregnancies were found to be comparable, but the C-section deliveries posed greater risk for the mother with no offsetting benefit for the baby.[14]

Many women are advised to have a C-section if they have had a C-section in a previous pregnancy. "Once a C-section, always a C-section" has been the gospel, followed religiously until recently. But the gospel is now disputed. The American College of

Obstetricians and Gynecologists opposes it, wants the practice changed. But so far they haven't succeeded. In spite of an increasing consensus among experts to let women try to deliver vaginally even if they've had a C-section (depending on the particular circumstances, of course), practitioners are not following the advice. "We're a bit disappointed but this is a tough thing to do. We're asking doctors to reverse a very longstanding practice," says Dr. Mort Lebow of the American College of Obstetricians and Gynecologists. There it is again—"style of practice" determining your fate instead of the best scientific evidence available!

What then would be the appropriate C-section rate for the United States? We don't know. According to the Public Citizens' Health Research Group study of the 1986 figures, the national rate of 24 percent should be cut in half, with rates as high as 17 percent at hospitals caring for high-risk pregnancies and as low as 7 percent in community hospitals with mostly low-risk patients. Dr. Warren Pearse, executive director of the American College of Obstetricians and Gynecologists, agrees that the present rate is too high. And increasingly we can, by taking charge, improve the likelihood of making the best decision for ourselves, in our particular circumstances.

The story of C-sections is a microcosm of how medicine is practiced in America. New technology is developed that enables us to do things we never could, to detect problems early, to surgically correct or avoid them. But the speed with which the technology is developed and put to use outstrips our capacity to evaluate its proper use or to understand its full implications. We use it as much as we can. We expand its limits. We push it to the hilt until slowly, over time, we learn from enough cases that we've pushed too far, that we've gone beyond solving old problems and are creating new and unnecessary ones. So use is cut back until, we hope, the appropriate level is found. For C-sections, there probably should be more than were done twenty years ago but fewer than are being done today. Trial and error: data becoming available bit by bit over time, experts making recommendations for change, practice patterns lagging behind. And in that interval, which can last for many years, whether you get the benefit of what is most currently known, or are limited by an outmoded style of practice, depends on your taking charge.

CANCER

Cancer. The very word strikes fear in the heart of everyone—and with good cause! In 1985 alone, more than 900,000 people heard the words "You have cancer" from their physicians. Over 450,000 American families buried a victim of cancer. We all know someone who has it, someone who has died from it. We have seen how slow and painful the process can be and how, in many instances, the treatments themselves can be a unique torture of their own. We have seen people "lick it," and we admire them as "special." For many of us, locked away in our secret consciousness is the fear that we might be next. How many of us have looked at a mole and wondered whether it was changing in size or color—could it be a melanoma? How many of us with a sore throat have felt swollen lymph nodes in our neck—could it be a lymphoma? How many of us have become convinced, without any real basis at all, that this year's physical will uncover something dreadfully wrong with us—a hidden cancer? And what words could cause us more pain than "Your child has cancer"?

Taking charge is particularly important if the disease is cancer. But the emotional shock of discovering that they have cancer leaves most people unusually vulnerable and dependent on the physician who makes the diagnosis, even though that physician may not be the best person or even the right person to manage the case. Most times that first physician will make the early decisions, even if it is only to choose another doctor to take over. But these early choices of physician and treatment can be the most important if the patient is going to have the best chance to get better. It's important to understand why you must take charge right from the start, and to understand why, we have to review the progress of the "War on Cancer," announced by President Nixon as one of our national goals.

Ever since the early 1970s, the War on Cancer has reflected a nationwide concern about the horrible toll of death and suffering from cancer, the widespread fear of cancer, and our very poor record in understanding and treating these diseases, much less preventing them.

Billions of dollars have been spent on the war, and in December 1985, the generals at the National Cancer Institute issued the following report:[1]

1. After the first ten years of battle, the chance of getting cancer in 1983 had increased over 1974 by a total of 6.3 percent.

2. More people died of cancer in 1983 than when the war began in 1974. In fact, the mortality rate went up 4.2 percent during the ten-year war.

3. The chances of surviving cancer without dying from it within five years increased slightly, from 48.5 percent to 49 percent.

To put these statistics another way, if the incidence of cancer, the mortality rate from cancer, and the five-year survival rate from cancer had all stayed the same in 1983 as they had been in 1974, 21,200 Americans would not have died. In other words, cancer had become a more deadly enemy between 1974 and 1983 in spite of all our efforts.

In most wars, generals who reported this kind of "progress" after ten years would be court-martialed. But the situation is not as bleak as it seems, nor is this the kind of war where ten years can or should be expected to produce a victory. The opportunities for any individual to influence the outcome in a cancer case successfully by taking charge are good, and they improve as you look beyond the broad statistics to individual cancer figures, beyond individual cancer statistics to specific treatments, beyond specific treatments to specific doctors and hospitals, beyond them to experimental therapies.

Let's look at where we stand on individual cancers: We know that the overall incidence of cancer in 1983 was higher than in 1974. But that is a composite figure. The incidence of some cancers went up, and some went down. For example, the incidence of colon and rectal cancer went up 4.7 percent; lung cancer in males went up 12.6 percent and in females 70 percent; non-Hodgkin's disease lymphomas went up 27.7 percent; melanomas 26.2 percent. But during the same ten years, the incidence of other cancers went down: leukemia by 8.3 percent; Hodgkin's disease by 13.8 percent; uterine cancer by 21.4 percent, and ovarian cancer by 7.9 percent. Yet with the exception of uterine cancer, the chances of living five years without being killed by the cancer have *increased for every disease.*

Lung cancer statistics have had the greatest impact on the overall progress of the war on cancer. Lung cancer is a true epidemic, a public health emergency. Treatment is ineffective. To conquer it depends not on the success of the generals and their scientists but on the actions of individuals. Prevention works, and the simple act of not smoking would reverse the tide of battle against this disease. In the battle against lung cancer, there are no true noncombatants. Everyone should become involved—to stop teenagers from smoking, to help friends and relatives to stop, to join the fight to get the government out of subsidizing tobacco industry support programs and more effectively into the fight to prevent this self-inflicted epidemic. Think of the millions of dollars that have been spent trying to hook young Americans on a deadly habit. For years on television, and still today in newspapers, magazines, billboards, and in the sponsoring of sports events, the unwitting modern-day merchants of death not only fight against public health measures, but they also deny that any serious problem exists. Taking charge is important in the fight against lung cancer because the opponent is more than the disease. It's an industry that uses all the tools of modern communication to keep the product that causes the disease as "American as apple pie."

How bad is this epidemic? In 1985, 125,600 Americans died of lung cancer, more than 25 percent of all cancer deaths combined, and another 144,000 Americans developed the disease. In the ten years of the war on cancer, the mortality rate for lung cancer has gone up 15.4 percent for males and 71.6 percent for females. Of all the major cancers, lung cancer has the poorest five-year relative survival rate: More than 88 out of every 100 men and 84 out of every 100 women will be dead within five years of getting this killer disease. If the disease merely acted in 1983 the way it acted in 1974, 25,800 more people would have lived to see 1984!

Can taking charge make a difference? You bet it can, and there's now definitive proof of the effectiveness of knowing the facts and making the decisions. White males have been smoking less, and as a group may have turned the corner in the war against lung cancer. In 1965, 52 percent of all white males of age twenty or more smoked. By March 1985, that figure had fallen to 30 percent. The incidence of lung cancer in white males dropped for the first time in a significant way—by 4.1 percent between 1982 and 1983. As a result, the 1983 rate has stayed equivalent to the 1977 rate. It has not grown by 60 percent, as it has for women. To put it simply, white males are smoking less than they used to and are hearing the dreaded words "You have lung cancer" less frequently than they used to. No such progress was made among white females or black males or females. For white males we may be seeing the light at the end of the tunnel, but it is a very, very long tunnel and there is no assurance that this favorable trend, which depends on continued progress in the effort to decrease smoking, will continue.

So profound is the impact of lung cancer on the overall status of the war on cancer that without those statistics figured in, the picture is quite different. There were 21,200 more deaths in 1983 than would have been expected from the 1974 cancer rates. If you take out lung cancer, there would have been 4,600 *fewer* than expected. Still a war far from over, still a war close to stalemate, but not a war with the disease advancing as dramatically.

The lung cancer epidemic marches on, but by breaking down the overall figures, we can see that one portion of the population—white males—is making some progress. Often the only way to detect such hidden progress is to examine how each population group fares. When it comes to cancer, all people are not created equal; blacks and whites, males and females fare differently in the battle against common cancers. In general, blacks do worse than whites. Blacks have a higher chance of getting cancer and a poorer rate of surviving five years with it. For many common cancers—uterine, breast, bladder, prostate, larynx, oral cavity and pharynx, rectum, and melanoma—the five-year survival rates for whites are more than *ten percentage points better* than for blacks. For other cancers—leukemia, cervix, lung, colon, and esophagus—there are smaller but still significantly better survival rates. In fact, whites have a statistically significant five-year survival rate advantage over blacks for thirteen of the twenty-four primary cancer sites. Although black survival is slightly better than that for whites for a few cancers—multiple myeloma, brain, kidney, ovary, and pancreas—in no case is the difference statistically significant.

What can account for the fact that blacks get more cancer than whites, and that they are killed more frequently by it? There are certainly many factors, but the major one may well be the basic inequality of life for whites and blacks in America. After all, black babies die at birth far more frequently than white babies. Blacks do not live as long, on the average, as whites. The legacy of racial discrimination still pervades every aspect of American society, and as a result, to be born black in America is to be born at a different starting line—one that is behind the white line. This has consequences in all walks of life, including income level, educational opportunity, employment possibilities, and health care. Blacks have a separate and unequal health care system in America, not by law, but by practice. This is why, by almost every measure of health status, they are statistically, at least, second-class citizens. There may be no organized conspiracy to keep it that way, but the disparities are woven into the very fabric of our society, and into the health care system itself. That is why change will be so slow.

When it comes to cancer, blacks pay dearly for their inequality. For many, a healthy diet may be beyond their pocketbooks and their education. The living environment may include far more numerous cancer risk factors. Early detection of disease is far less likely because visits to physicians, in the absence of serious illness, are less frequent, and the facilities where the already delayed treatment is sought may not be of adequate quality.

Taking charge is important for all cancer patients, but it is particularly important for blacks. If your disease is caught late, your chances of survival are less, and the importance of taking charge is greater. Just as blacks do worse than whites, it is also true that males do worse than females—black or white. In the first ten years of the war on cancer, the chance of getting cancer increased most rapidly for black males. White males were next, then black females, and finally white females.

Although the results of the first ten years of the war on cancer are discouraging when looked at overall, and are worse for blacks than for whites, some individual battles have gone well. Taking charge depends less on what is happening in the overall war than on the particular disease one is battling at the time. It requires not only advocacy, but informed advocacy, based on what you can and should know about the disease you or your friend might have. The history of breast cancer shows the urgency of taking charge very clearly.

Breast cancer makes a good example because the overall statistics are very gloomy despite scientific advances and lots of publicity. Treatments have been radically altered over the years, but with little effect on outcome. Nonetheless, for this disease, taking charge can result in saving thousands of lives that would otherwise be lost.

The sad, overwhelming fact is that survival of breast cancer patients has not improved at all since the war on cancer began. It makes no difference whether the patient is under or over age fifty, or whether she was diagnosed in 1974 or 1983. And as usual, blacks fare worse than whites.

Over the years, treatments for breast cancer have come in and out of favor and have caused great controversy. Each new treatment has been announced as "the answer," and yet the statistics show that "the answer" is not yet clear. But the consequences to the patient of the various approaches vary enormously. For more than three quarters of a century, mutilating surgery was performed, unnecessarily it now turns out, on thousands and thousands of women. The so-called Halsted technique, developed by Johns Hopkins surgeon William Halsted in the late nineteenth century, was a veritable nightmare for the patient. She would lose her entire breast, the underlying chest muscles, and have the armpit surgically dissected so that all the lymph nodes could be found and removed. Halsted claimed remarkable results from this procedure and publicly pronounced that breast cancer was a potentially curable disease. Even though few, if any, surgeons ever replicated Halsted's phenomenal results, and even though the failure to replicate them was publicly reported by a number of other physicians, the Halsted procedure took hold and became the law.[2]

Once something gets widely accepted by the medical community, it can take a very long time to undo it, no matter how wrong it is! It was more than fifty years before the tide began to turn against the procedure. The turn was inevitable because the disease wasn't cured, and the results of individual surgeons were not consistent with Halsted's. We now know of the basic scientific fallacy underlying the Halsted approach to all breast cancer: He believed that it spread outward from its original location on a steady, predictable route much like a train moving along an uninterrupted track. If a large portion of the track—up to the nodes in the armpit—were removed, he believed, then the disease could be cured. Only if the disease had traveled beyond that area would the procedure fail. Because one can't see cancer with the naked eye, one has to take a large section of track. Better to be safe than sorry. Mutilation is a small price to pay for survival. Sound reasoning. But wrong! It is now believed that breast cancer does not spread contiguously, but can skip sections of "track" and appear somewhere else. This was suspected as early as the 1930s, but had little immediate impact on slowing down radical surgery as the treatment of choice for all breast cancer.

In fact, even when science dictates a change in approach to a disease, there is usually a lag time before the change is incorporated into the daily practice of the preponderance of physicians. During this lag, the treatment a patient receives is dependent more on whose door she walks through than on the best current knowledge of the disease. This is where taking charge is critical, because in such circumstances only you or your advocate can take steps to assure that you are presented with the full range of existing treatment options. The fact that your doctor prefers one approach may be based on habit, on ignorance, or on an irrational personal conviction. But it is you who must undergo the treatment and pay the price if it is not the best available treatment. Often there is no best, and you must choose among competing alternatives, each with strengths and weaknesses. But in many instances, there is a best treatment. You may have to find it out for yourself instead of accepting the word of a physician who simply may not know what else is available.

What is the status of breast cancer treatment today? For one thing the debate between advocates of conservative surgery and radical surgery goes on. The most celebrated modern debaters are Thomas J. Anglem of Boston and George Crile, Jr., of Cleveland. Women who go to Dr. Anglem may be more likely to have radical surgery than those going to Dr. Crile. For another, it is generally accepted that surgery is not the only tool available. Radiation therapy, chemotherapy, and hormonal therapy are also part of the arsenal.

Today we know that there are different forms of breast cancer, and we classify them by different cell types. But these categories have a small influence on prognosis or choice of treatment. A large influence is exerted by how early the disease is detected; the age, menopausal status, and general health of the patient; as well as some technical characteristics of the tumor itself. Breast cancer is generally classified into five categories, and unlike in the old days, the treatment of each category is approached differently. Noninvasive local cancer is called breast cancer *in situ*, or Category 1. The next Category is called Stage I breast cancer, followed by Stage II breast cancer, Stage III breast cancer, and Stage IV breast cancer. Noninvasive breast cancer is the most curable; Stage IV breast cancer is the least curable.

These are important facts to know. Why? Because you must be sure you know all the treatment options for each stage. These options are constantly revised as new information becomes available. For example, the National Cancer Institute acknowledges that the "customary treatment" for noninvasive breast cancer has been mastectomy plus the removal of some lymph nodes in the armpit. Yet the institute also points out that "limited resection of breast tissue provides the diagnosis and is curative."[3] Although its study of limited breast cancer surgery is still in progress, and, therefore, the recommended approach may be modified by the time you read this book, as of this writing the institute lists *four* treatment options as standard—ranging from lumpectomy all the way to the "customary" treatment, total mastectomy and removal of armpit lymph nodes. The better-safe-than-sorry theory doesn't necessarily hold true: "Limited experience with conservative surgery and radiation therapy suggests that local control with this approach is acceptable and overall survival excellent."

Four standard options—but only one patient. Taking charge can make the difference between having the "customary" procedure or considering instead a much less radical but potentially equally effective approach. Your doctor may recommend the customary approach because he is unaware of the alternatives, because he is used to his own approach, or because he is skeptical of other treatments. In any particular case, he may be right or wrong, but it is not his decision to make alone. Taking charge means making sure that an informed choice is made among the alternatives, and refusing to accept a recommendation with as far-reaching consequences as radical surgery without probing for alternatives.

The same range of alternatives exists for other stages of breast cancer. Stage I breast cancer, in the Halsted days, would have been treated with mutilating surgery. Today, according to the National Cancer Institute, "Stage I breast cancer is *highly curable* with a *range of surgical procedures*. Surgical procedures which *conserve a major portion of the involved breast* followed by radiotherapy *provide tumor control equivalent to more extensive surgical procedures* [emphasis added]." There are times when the more radical surgical approach is the appropriate one, even for Stage I treatment, but certainly not for the majority of Stage I cases; certainly not as the routine procedure; certainly not without performing the appropriate laboratory tests to confirm its necessity. The Cancer Institute officially tells physicians, "It is then appropriate to discuss the therapeutic options of mastectomy versus conservative surgery and radiation therapy to help the patient with the treatment decision." And, as the Institute also makes clear, the patient's feelings about the procedure are a legitimate component of the decision-making process: "Selection of the appropriate therapeutic approach depends on the location and size of the lesion, breast size, and whether the patient feels *strongly about preservation of the breast* [emphasis added]."

Under the treatment options for physicians, the Cancer Institute lists four:

1. A lumpectomy with armpit node dissection and radiotherapy.

2. A partial breast resection with lymph node dissection and radiotherapy.

3. A modified radical or total mastectomy.

4. A radical mastectomy, which should be used, according to the report, "in highly selected circumstances only if needed to accomplish complete tumor resection locally."

We have obviously come a long way from Halsted's approach to all breast cancer! The official U.S. government spearhead of the war on cancer urges consideration of far more conservative options, and recognizes the patient's feelings about saving the breast as a legitimate decision-making factor.

In America today, two women with equivalent Stage I cancers walking into different doctors' offices might get very different advice, very different degrees of choice, and very different treatments. One might get mutilating surgery and the other a very limited local excision of the lump. Yet both approaches in this hypothetical example would have an equivalent chance of cure. If someone was taking charge, the full range of options would be considered before a decision was reached. Equally important, the method of presenting the alternatives would not bias the decision in advance. If a physician has a strong preference, whether based on experience, fact, or prejudice, it can affect the way the patient's choice is presented. By taking charge, you recognize that possibility and compensate for it. You can select consultants and use the other sources of information we will discuss (see page 164) to assure a full and impartial disclosure of all known options. The patient with Stage I breast cancer has several potentially good options short of extensive surgery. Whether she learns about them depends in part on where she lives and which doctor she sees, but also on whether she or someone close to her is taking charge.

Options short of radical surgery also exist for the more extensive Stage II breast cancer. According to the National Cancer Institute, "Stage II breast cancer is curable *with a range of accepted surgical procedures. Conservative surgical approaches which salvage a portion of the breast* followed by postoperative radiation therapy can provide tumor control *equivalent to more extensive surgery* [emphasis added]." Again, for Stage II breast cancer the patient's feelings "about preservation of the breast" are considered important. Can all extensive surgery for Stage II breast cancer be avoided? No, of course not. But in many instances it can be, and without diminishing the chance for success of the treatment. Although the overall treatment of Stage II breast cancer is more complex than for Stage I, the surgical options remain the same, and the same caution to use radical mastectomy *"in selected circumstances only"* is advised by the National Cancer Institute.

Stage III breast cancer is far more serious and must be classified into operable and nonoperable cases. Here the surgical options are far more limited—modified radical or full radical mastectomy. Radiation, chemotherapy, and hormonal therapy treatments can also be used, either separately or together.

Stage IV breast cancer is the most advanced, with "durable complete remissions" obtainable in only 10 percent to 20 percent of patients. Here the role of surgery is quite limited. The cancer is so advanced that there is no point in surgery, either for therapy or for diagnostic biopsies. Radical breast surgery stands alone as the treatment of choice today *only* for Stage III breast cancer.

Despite the wide range of treatment options available today for breast cancer patients, we must still face up to perhaps the most important reality of all: In spite of much new knowledge about breast cancer, in spite of our ability to identify it more precisely and to fine-tune a given treatment to a given stage, in spite of the development of many new drugs and radiotherapy techniques, the fact is that overall survival of patients with the disease has not improved since the war on cancer began. Why? We don't know all the answers, but we do know one. Breast cancer is simply not being detected as early as it should be, or as it could be.

The basic fact about breast cancer is very simple: The earlier it is detected, the easier it is to cure. We have a way to detect breast cancer early—mammography, which provides so clear an X ray of the breast that an experienced radiologist can usually detect the smallest tumor. A study sponsored by the American Cancer Society reported in September 1987 the astonishing success of mammography in reducing breast cancer fatalities in women in their forties and older. The study, which covered more than 280,000 women for up to eleven years, clearly showed the value of routine mammography screening: 4,240 cases of breast cancer were detected so early, before the tumors could be felt by normal breast examination, that the tumors could usually be removed with lumpectomy surgery. The survival rate was an impressive 88 percent after five years, 83 percent after eight years, and 79 percent after ten years. These survival rates are significantly better than the Cancer Institute's figures: 74 percent survival after five years, and 65 percent after eight years.

We simply aren't using mammography, however. We're not using it for many reasons. Most insurers don't pay for mammography as a screening test, doctors don't recommend it often enough, and patients are not taking charge and demanding it. Those who do have to pay between $75 and $150—a worthwhile expense for women over thirty-five to discuss with their doctors.

If we have not made overall progress in the battle against breast cancer, it is at least in part because we are finding the disease too late. New treatments may reduce the critical importance of early detection, but in the meantime, the real progress that can be made will depend more on individuals demanding mammography than on the fruits of laboratory research. It is clear from what we now know that the doctors won't adequately push you to be screened. So you must push them.

Here are the startling facts as presented by Dr. Peter Greenwald, the director of cancer prevention and control for the National Cancer Institute, in a 1986 speech: The death rate from breast cancer *could be reduced nearly a third by early detection with mammography.* In spite of this, only 11 percent of doctors are recommending that this proven life-saving test be carried out, and only 15 percent of women over the age of fifty have had at least one mammogram. The remaining eighty-five out of every one hundred women over the age of fifty have failed to take the minimal steps necessary to reduce the risk of death from breast cancer. Yet the American Cancer Society recommends a mammogram every year for women over fifty and every other year for women between the ages of forty and fifty. Women at particularly high risk of the disease—those with breast cancer in the immediate family—might need to follow a different, more rigorous screening process.

Taking charge is necessary when obtaining medical care because the quality of physicians varies, their knowledge about particular diseases varies, their knowledge about new treatments varies, and they bring certain biases and convictions to the treatment of particular diseases. By taking charge, you can challenge those biases and get them out in the open for evaluation. As a result, you have a much better chance of reviewing all the treatment options, especially the most current ones, and of bringing the most accurate information about a disease to bear on the case.

How would that work in this example? Dr. Greenwald points to three major reasons for the inexcusable underuse of mammography:

1. One third of doctors assert that they are not convinced of its value. Here, by taking charge you would confront the doctor with the strong recommendations of both the National Cancer Institute and the American Cancer Society. What does your doctor know that these generals in the war on cancer don't? Taking charge can at least force your doctor to confront the evidence, to look it up. Your doctor's bias against the procedure must be based on more than intuition, more than simply "not being convinced of its value." After all, it's your life, not your physician's, that is at risk by following bad advice.

2. One fifth of physicians don't recommend mammography explicitly because of fears of radiation exposure for the patient.

By taking charge, you would point out to your doctor that the American College of Radiology defines the risk from mammograms for women aged forty and over as negligible—not a factor at all. Again, what does your doctor know that these experts don't? What is his evidence? How does it compare with that of the College of Radiology? What is the magnitude of the risk as he sees it? Whose risk is it anyway? Should he decide for you, or should you decide for yourself? Even if you have never heard of the College of Radiology, you can ask who recommends mammograms, why they do, and what results have been obtained. If your doctor can't answer these questions, have him find out—or get a new doctor!

3. One third of physicians worry about financial reimbursement for the test because insurers may not pay for screening tests in apparently healthy women. But this is a financial consideration, made by a doctor, with potentially profound health consequences for the patient. By taking charge, you would tell your doctor to separate medical advice from economic concern. It is your decision whether to pay out of your pocket for this procedure. It is his responsibility to make it clear, in advance, that you may have to. Taking charge in this instance has an additional dimension. It is a scandal that a screening test for breast cancer which can save over ten thousand lives a year is not paid for in some insurance policies and therefore may not be recommended by doctors or may be out of reach of women who later die from a breast cancer that could have been detected earlier. This is something state regulators can correct. Write them!

How effective can taking charge be in the early detection of breast cancer? Very. There is no substitute for it. If you need more convincing, consider this: In 1974, the wives of the President and Vice President of the United States—Betty Ford and Happy Rockefeller—both developed breast cancer. There was an avalanche of publicity at the time, and in effect thousands of women across America, motivated by that publicity, descended on their doctors to be examined for breast cancer. For that brief period, the incidence of breast cancer in America rose 14 percent—a statistically astounding figure. Of course, more women did not suddenly get cancer; more cancer was found, and found early in the disease. As a result of this nationwide effort at taking charge, the cases diagnosed in this period appear to have a significantly increased survival rate over those diagnosed earlier that same year, before the publicity. Two years later, with the publicity gone, cases were once again being detected at later stages, and the survival rates dropped back to the prepublicity levels. Nancy Reagan's cancer may awaken public awareness once again.

Diagnosing breast cancer before it becomes too advanced is critically important, but no matter how widespread the use of mammography becomes, many women will still come to their doctors for treatment of advanced-stage disease. In these cases, taking charge can literally mean the difference between life and death, or at least between longer, high-quality life and early death. In medicine generally, the more complicated the problem, or the more advanced the disease, the more important it is to find the right doctor. Almost all doctors can handle routine problems. Almost all can handle hopeless cases—those for which no treatment exists—with equal compassion. But in the vast middle ground, where the bulk of serious cases fall, the choice of doctor can make a profound difference. New drugs, new combinations of drugs, new hormonal therapies, new forms of radiation treatments develop constantly in the field of cancer treatment. Some work; some don't. The state of the art is constantly changing, not only in therapies but in diagnostic tests.

The treatment of cancer is a recognized medical specialty in and of itself. Even so, one individual spending a lifetime treating only cancer patients could not possibly stay on top of all the new information. As a result, there are subspecialties within the specialty of cancer. Some doctors are particular experts in Hodgkin's disease, or leukemia, or colorectal cancer, or breast cancer.

Very few people with a complicated cancer can walk into the office of a national expert on that problem. Most people with cancer, between 80 percent and 85 percent, walk through the doors of their community physician. On the whole, these are hardworking, dedicated frontline physicians, but they don't see only cancer patients; they see virtually every kind of medical problem. They can't possibly know about every disease. The best of them know their limitations, know when to ask for help. The fact is, however, that walking through the door of a community physician's office to have cancer diagnosed and treated is a game of Russian roulette.

Are we exaggerating the problem? Hardly. According to the chief general of the nation's war on cancer, Dr. Vincent De Vita, director of the National Cancer Institute, cancer should be curable in *half* the patients with serious tumors![4] But De Vita points out that achieving this cure rate requires that patients have access to the best available therapy. Where is that "best therapy" available? Because developments occur so rapidly in this field, the best therapies are usually available in research centers, in university hospitals. But few patients get to those centers, or can expect to get to them under the present system. Most people are seen by community physicians who may or may not be up to date or capable of giving the best therapy. According to De Vita, "The greatest problem for these doctors is keeping up." It may be the greatest problem for the doctors. It is even greater for the patient who pays for this failure with his life.

To cope with this potentially life-threatening information gap between what is known to be the best and what is actually utilized in the community physician's office, the National Cancer Institute has developed a national, computer-based information system called *PDQ* (*Physician Data Query*). Learn those initials. They may save your life. All your physician needs to link up to the system is a personal computer. *PDQ* contains detailed information on the prognosis, staging procedures, and known treatments for all major diseases. It also alerts your doctor to ongoing experimental treatments for which you may be eligible. It lists specialists to whom your doctor can turn for help.

If all physicians used *PDQ*, the best and latest information would be available to them, and the great national cancer information gap would be closed. Make sure your doctor reviews all the information in *PDQ* before discussing options. If he has never heard of *PDQ*, tell him about it! If he doesn't belong, make him get the information from a colleague's computer. If he won't, or if he says he knows it all already (even though he hasn't heard of *PDQ*), change doctors.

But you should be able to do more than tell him about *PDQ*. You should be able to show him what it can do. On page 225 you will find the full text of the *PDQ* "state-of-the-art information" on breast cancer as of January 27, 1988—the date the computer was queried. Take this book with you to your doctor and show him what *PDQ* can do. The *PDQ* may be different today, to reflect the newest information available. That is its virtue: It's always up to date.

Will doctors use this system? No one knows. Left to their own devices, few doctors may take advantage of *PDQ*. But if enough

Americans with cancer are taking charge, then *PDQ* will be used and the information gap can be closed dramatically.

Having access to the best and latest information is important, but it is only as meaningful as the use to which the information is put. For many doctors, the data will convince them to seek the help of a consultant. For others, it may make effective treatment in their own offices possible.

The fact is, however, that although a doctor may know what should be done, he may not do it anyway. Having information and understanding information do not always translate into using information well. Consider the following case. Harriet Jones* was a vigorous and athletic seventy-two-year-old woman living in California. The mother of a powerful, prominent son, she was used to and could afford the best of everything. When she noticed a swollen lymph node and went for evaluation, her doctor diagnosed cancer. Her form of cancer is not an easy one to treat, but it does have a reasonable chance for cure. She was referred to a well-known cancer specialist, who started her on the appropriate chemotherapy. For those who have never had it or known people undergoing chemotherapy, it is difficult to imagine how unpleasant the side effects can be—not for all cancer drugs, not to the same degree in every patient. But in many instances, it is an experience you would rather skip, and one whose memory can bring shudders years later to those who have gone through it.

Sometimes the side effects are life-threatening and difficult to treat. The process is not only hard on the patient; it can be hard on the doctor as well. It is hard emotionally for the doctor to inflict the misery, and it can be hard economically because the severe side effects often lead to malpractice suits.

*The names of all patients have been changed to protect their anonymity.

So chemotherapy can be unpleasant; it can be painful; it can be almost a form of torture. It can be one other thing as well: It can be a lifesaver, but only when used properly. And it wasn't used properly for Harriet Jones. She was given the chemotherapy; she suffered the expected side effects. And when the doctor saw the discomfort, and saw the pain of the treatment, he reduced the subsequent doses. When you lower the doses, however, you lower the effectiveness, and thus the chance for cure.

So Harriet Jones had chemotherapy. She had side effects. And she had a relapse, a recurrence. What she never had was the chance that taking charge would have made possible: the chance to consider her options and make her own decision. She, or her advocate, could have weighed the discomfort of the therapy against the chance of a recurrence of her disease. In general, once a cancer recurs, the chance of successful treatment is reduced. With each recurrence, the chance for success drops further.

Harriet Jones is not unique. According to Dr. De Vita, as many as *nine thousand patients may die each year because they receive too low a dose of an otherwise effective chemotherapy.*[5] Even small reductions in dosage significantly reduce a treatment's effectiveness, in his opinion. Why are doctors doing it? Dr. William Hryniuk, of McMaster University in Ontario, Canada, studied this problem and gave two reasons: the adverse side effects of the treatments, and the fear of malpractice suits.

How many patients would opt to have their dosages of chemotherapy reduced if they knew the profound effect the reduction would have on their chances for a cure? How many patients are even asked?

The fact is that cancer kills. Left untreated, most cancers kill most of the time. Most ineffectively treated cancers also kill most of the time. When you fight against cancer, you fight for your life, for a cure. If that is not possible, you fight for time, quality time—as much as you can get.

When you fight a killer, you fight hard. In the war on cancer, many of the treatments make you sick, much sicker than the disease itself may have made you up to that point. But you have to know that going in, because you are fighting for your life.

When is it appropriate to cut back doses? When they produce life-threatening effects that can't be managed if the treatment continues. Or when you decide you've had enough and the cost of the fight is no longer worth paying. When you decide, not when your doctor decides for you. Not when your doctor, without consultation, decides to spare you the terrible side effects without telling you the consequences. And certainly not when he fears a malpractice suit.

Perhaps some doctors stop because they feel they can't adequately treat the life-threatening side effects. In that case, you should change doctors before changing dosages. For once that dose is reduced, once the treatment becomes less effective, once the killer escapes, you don't get another equally good chance. There may be another doctor who would be able to cope with the side effects.

The best cancer doctors are those who push known and experimental treatments to their limits, who can effectively manage side effects and not be scared off by them, and who do all this with the informed consent of the patient. Even the best, most experienced cancer doctors sometimes have to lower dosages or even stop treatment because of side effects. But many others stop too soon, before they have to.

Not all patients will want their treatment pushed to the limit. The point is that it's your decision. There is no right or wrong. There are facts about the disease to be known, facts about treat-

ment alternatives to be known. But there are also quality-of-life—
current life—considerations to be made. Different people with
the same disease and the same treatment options may make
different decisions. But they must be *your* decisions. You can
make them with your doctor's help, but they must be made by
you because you will have to live—or die—with the consequences.

The success of chemotherapy can often depend more on the
choice of doctor than on the disease. It's hard to believe that the
mere act of walking through a given doctor's door, or into a
particular hospital, can so profoundly affect your chance for a
cure, but it does. And there are many examples. In 1982, the
American Cancer Society reported in its journal, *Cancer*, the
startling findings of a study of the treatment of brain tumors in
children in the state of Connecticut. All parents, no matter what
state they live in, should know what these researchers found:
Where the children received treatment turned out to make an
enormous difference in whether they lived or died from certain
forms of cancer. For children with one form of disease, treated
at a university cancer center, the projected five-year survival rate
was 74 percent; but for other children with the same disease, who
were treated at community hospitals, the projected five-year survival rate was 29 percent. Seventy-four percent versus 29 percent!
The difference was the place, not the disease. For a second form
of brain cancer, children treated in university cancer centers had
projected five-year survival rates of 40 percent; but of children
treated for the same disease in community hospitals, only one
child was alive thirteen months after the diagnosis.[6]

The outcome did not vary with the place of treatment for all
forms of brain cancer in children. For hopeless cases, where no
known treatment is effective, the place made no difference. For

simpler cases, where surgery alone was sufficient for cure, the place made no difference. But for the complex cases, where proven but complicated mixtures of surgical, chemical, and radiation therapies are required, the place can make a dramatic difference.

The same differences were demonstrated in a study in the treatment of a different childhood cancer—Wilms' tumor—in upstate New York. Between 1967 and 1972, those patients treated in the Buffalo area had a seven-year survival rate of 87 percent. Children with the same disease, treated in the less populous counties outside Buffalo, had a 50 percent seven-year survival rate. Same disease; different places of treatment. If it's your child, that's a big difference. The authors of this study attributed the difference to "the better treatment and care available at some of the hospitals in Buffalo."[7]

Variations in the quality of radiation therapy, variations that dramatically affect the chance for a cure, have been reported repeatedly in *Cancer*. One such study in 1985 showed that the equipment being used, the way it was used, and the skill and experience of the person using it were directly related to the success of the treatment of Hodgkin's disease, prostate cancer, and cancer of the cervix.[8] If you had one of these diseases and walked through the door of a facility using a certain type of equipment—a less than 80 cm cobalt unit—chances are 75 percent that you were treated by a part-time practitioner. The combination of part-time practitioners and less than adequate equipment would seriously reduce your chances for proper treatment. This study found such facilities to have "poor technical support and exhibit poor staging, poor achievement of minimum tumor dose and poor patient follow-up." The study concluded,

"These facilities should either upgrade their equipment, technical support, and level of practice or close."

But until the facilities do so, taking charge is required to be sure you avoid them. There are no "grades" posted anywhere, no directory where you can find doctors or hospitals ranked by quality. The only way to find out where to go is by asking the right questions, getting the right information, seeking the right consultations—by taking charge.

Let's look at one of the great successes in the war on cancer, the treatment of Hodgkin's disease. Deaths from Hodgkin's disease have declined by 43 percent in the first ten years of the war on cancer. But it could be more. When radiation therapy is used, the cure depends in large part on the precision with which the radiation is delivered. Even at university medical centers that precision varies, and with those variations come very different results. For example, in one study of patients treated only with radiation, there was a 54 percent overall relapse rate when the radiation was not properly delivered, compared with a 14 percent relapse rate when it was.[9] Fifty-four percent versus 14 percent—same disease, different quality treatments. The authors of this study concluded that, in the treatment of Hodgkin's disease, "marked facility differences exist in this technical process, and . . . skilled independent observers can reliably identify inaccurate technical performance." To put it bluntly: Competence varies, and people can pay for the variation with their lives. We know how to deliver the radiation appropriately; it is a technical job. The track record can be monitored and improved. But there is no compulsory system for doing so. According to the authors of the study, "These data in Hodgkin's disease provide further evidence of the need for an individual facility evaluation of the practice of radiation therapy to determine *where this high-tech-*

nology disease is being most adequately treated. Clearly, facilities that do not have the technical support for these complex treatment programs should *not be involved* in the curative management of Hodgkin's disease [emphasis added]."

How do you find out where to go? By taking charge, as we describe it in the last section of this book.

Equally dramatic findings of wide variations in quality have been reported for the radiation treatment of cancer of the cervix.[10] The authors of the study found a "substantial variation . . . from a consensus of best current management." By almost all criteria, part-time practitioners, small facilities, and freestanding facilities ranked below the national average. University centers, large facilities, and doctors specializing in cancer radiation therapy ranked consistently above the national average. If you have cancer of the cervix, Stage IIIB, for example, the difference can be very serious. The national average for control of this form of the disease is only 28 percent. The best large facilities can control 60 percent. Twenty-eight percent versus 60 percent— same disease, different quality of care. The authors who studied this disease concluded, "If we cannot bring the national average to the level of these large facilities, then *all patients* with advanced cervical cancer should be treated in facilities with large annual experience and *proven success* in cancer of the cervix [emphasis added]."

Do we know how to bring the other institutions up to the top standard? Yes. But evolution in medicine is slow. There is a lag between finding what works and implementing it throughout the system. Sometimes the lag can last for many, many years, and improvements at your hospital won't help you if they come after you've been unsuccessfully treated. By taking charge you can find the best current treatment available—before you go through it.

. . .

We know that the overall statistics of the first ten years of the war on cancer are disappointing. We know that there are specific examples of progress against some diseases, and examples of failure for others. But the figures by which we measure progress, or lack of it, are overall figures. Behind each of these statistics are human beings, and it is from the overall aggregate experience of these individual cancer patients that the statistics are composed. When the statistics indicate progress against a certain disease, there are still many, many cancer patients who lose their individual battles. When the statistics indicate lack of progress, there are still many individuals who win their personal battles. For every cancer there are winners and losers, no matter what the overall statistical odds are. Taking charge is one way to improve the chances of winning the individual battle.

There is another factor to consider. If new treatments are developed this year which prove to be extremely effective against breast cancer, that progress will not be apparent in the statistics for several years, perhaps as many as five to ten years. That is because a new treatment will not affect the incidence of the disease. The mortality figures will include primarily those people who developed the disease years before the new treatment was available and may now be beyond its reach. And the five-year survival figures obviously have no validity for the new treatment until the five years have passed. Thus the overall statistics are a benchmark, a guide to the relative power of the disease. They are not an indicator of any individual's chances. Each cancer patient must fight to become a success story. Taking charge cannot assure victory but it can assure the best opportunity for it. Sometimes the disease is just too powerful and nothing can change the outcome. But if you have cancer, and if you are going to lose the fight, it ought to be because of the inherent strength of your particular disease, and not because of the failings of your medical care. We have seen how variable that care can be: how access to the latest information varies widely, how experience with complicated cases varies widely, how information may not be used appropriately, how some doctors shy away from difficult but treatable side effects more quickly than others.

There is one other variable as well. Some doctors give up on their complicated cases more quickly than others. This is not a difference between community physicians and university-trained cancer specialists. It is a difference between individual doctors. Some of the most pronounced differences are among cancer specialists. Most of these doctors would quarrel with the phrase "giving up." They would argue that knowing when to stop, when there's nothing further to be done, when to let the patient maximize the time left, is an important element of the best medical treatment. That is true. But no matter how you package it, it is giving up. It may be right; it may be wrong. That is certainly debatable. What is not debatable is that it leads to certain death. And because of that, giving up should not be the doctor's decision alone. It is your decision, or that of your advocate, and is an important part of taking charge.

Consider this example. John Fox, a prominent sixty-four-year-old investment banker in Los Angeles, is involved in some of the most important and complicated financial transactions in America. Today, as this is written, he is fully active, at the peak of his power and influence. He is also in his ninth year after the discovery of colon cancer. During that time he has had several recurrences and has been operated on five times, each occasion a major surgery. Many of the nation's finest doctors and institutions have been involved in his case. With each succeeding recurrence and each succeeding operation, the debate among his doctors about what to do "the next time," for the next recurrence, has intensified. Statistically, John Fox is already a success in the war against cancer. He has lived longer and overcome more recurrences than most patients. Before the past several surgeries, some of his doctors argued forcefully against the treatment. The cancer would recur, they argued, and how much surgery can you put yourself through? they asked. What will you do if it recurs? they asked. Don't torture yourself, they argued. In effect, they were saying, "You've done well, you can have quality time left even without surgery. Give it up."

Many patients would have. But not John Fox. He listened, and he agonized, and he sought other opinions. He took charge. For him, the surgery was not torture. It was unpleasant, to be sure. But he always bounced back quickly. Surgery, in his mind, was not a barrier to "going for the cure." It was certainly no reason to give up. He wanted to do all he could, for as long as he could, to win the war. Some of his doctors just shook their heads, but John Fox had his surgeries and returned to a full and vigorous schedule after each one.

Right for everybody? No, of course not. But right for John Fox. Not many other patients would have stood up to nationally recognized experts and rejected their advice. But when it comes to giving up, their expertise is no match for yours, if you are the patient. How much you can take, how much you want to take, and for what purpose—that is up to you.

To make an intelligent decision, you must get a lot of information from your doctor, as John Fox did. The doctor can, with the best of motives, influence that decision with what he presents to you and how he presents it. By taking charge, you can help eliminate that bias. It is well known inside the medical profession that there are "aggressive treaters" and more conservative ones— a full spectrum can be found. The advice you get, the treatment you get, will depend on where your doctor falls on that spectrum.

The aggressive treater is the last to give up. "Foolish" is how someone at the other end of the spectrum would describe him—needlessly impairing the patient's quality of life through difficult treatments with minimal chances for success. Looked at the other way, the conservative treater would be called "foolish"—giving up when there is still a chance, or a new experimental treatment to be tried that might, just might, save the patient's life. After all, the aggressive treater argues, this is a life-or-death struggle. Use everything you've got.

Neither approach is invariably right or wrong, but they are different, with different consequences for you. You need to know that the differences exist, and to make your own decision. Sometimes that decision involves charting a course into the unknown, into the world of experimental treatments. There is a point in the lives of many gravely ill cancer patients who are to lose their individual battles when even the most aggressive treater will say, "We've tried everything that's known and nothing has worked." That's when a consideration of ongoing experimental treatments becomes relevant. We are not talking about the patient ravaged with disease, terminally ill and too weak to undergo any treatment. We are talking about patients who may feel well, but whose disease is advancing in spite of trying all known treatments. For these patients, taking charge means finding out what experimental treatments are being studied and where, and seeing whether they are appropriate to the particular case. When all that is known fails, you can take charge by seeking the answers at the frontiers of medicine. This is a long shot, but occasionally it works.

Take the case of Teddy Kennedy, Jr.: At age twelve, without warning, and with everything in the world ahead of him, he developed a deadly form of cancer—a mixed cancer of cartilage and bone. When his parents learned the diagnosis, they also heard the horrifying prognosis: Eighty-five percent of all children with his disease would die within five years. But by taking charge, his father learned of an experimental treatment that had been tried on just two other children. Teddy Jr. lost his leg to surgery and his hair, temporarily, to chemotherapy. But he gained his life. And that experimental treatment means that today 85 percent of all children with the disease are cured.

It was not wealth and power that made this possible for Teddy Jr. It was his father's taking charge. What Senator Kennedy did was to gather information about ongoing experimental treatments. Anyone can do the same by following the suggestions in the third part of this book. The decision to enter an experimental treatment is often a difficult one. At the outset, no one knows whether it will work. The extent of side effects is not known. Sometimes the doctors don't even know the right dosages or frequency of dosages. In an experimental protocol the primary purpose is to find out about the new treatment, not to cure the particular individual. In effect, you are the guinea pig from whose experience the doctors have to learn enough to help others effectively in the future. Cure is always hoped for, but is only a happy by-product to the researchers. Information gathering, learning what works and what doesn't, is the primary purpose. Because of this, many diagnostic and laboratory tests are done more for science than for an individual's treatment. Some patients have died in these experiments. Many have seen their disease resist the new treatments. And some have been cured or seen their disease go into remission.

An easy decision to undergo an experimental treatment? No. A pleasant experience? Rarely. Does it offer hope? Yes, but hope that is not frequently realized. Is it useful for scientists and a contribution to future generations? Almost always. But it is not for everybody. Again, it is your decision to make. You must know whether experimental treatments for your particular problem exist and what they entail, then make your own evaluation.

For many, experimental treatments represent the last chance, either for a cure or to gain quality time. For others, they may represent another round of doctor-induced illness for too little chance of success, at the cost of the precious quality time left. Only the patient can decide.

Developments in cancer research are occurring so rapidly today, and new approaches seem so promising, that playing for time is more important than ever. When going for a cure no longer seems possible, it may be worthwhile to try for slowing the disease down, arresting its progress, treating life-threatening metastases. If there is a breakthrough, if seemingly uncurable cases become curable at least some of the time, then taking charge can help you be around to take advantage of it. Again, this approach is not for everyone, but it is an option that should not be discarded for you by others. It is your choice.

In the final analysis, the war against cancer is a series of individual battles. The strategy in each case must be personalized. The crucial strategic decisions include which doctor to go to, which hospital to be treated in if necessary, which treatments to submit to, how many alternatives to try, whether experimental approaches are appropriate, and when to stop. Sometimes there are many pathways to a successful result. Sometimes choosing the right pathway makes the difference; sometimes no pathway works. The responsibility for choosing a pathway is yours. You can and should be guided by your physicians. But as this chapter has attempted to show, you cannot abdicate this responsibility and still have the best chance for a cure. There is simply no substitute for taking charge.

HEART DISEASE
AND HIGH BLOOD PRESSURE

John Henderson could not believe what had happened to him. On Tuesday he played an early morning set of tennis, as he had almost every morning for ten years. He felt great. On his way to the office, he stopped in for his routine physical examination, as he always did in the month before his birthday. And today, Monday, six days later, he was in the hospital recovery room. Earlier that morning, a team of skilled doctors and nurses had opened his chest, stopped his heart from beating while a mechanical heart-lung pump filled in, and replaced his diseased coronary arteries with veins that had been removed from his leg. He'd felt perfect before the surgery. He ached now.

His physical exam had shown an abnormal electrocardiogram. Because of this, the doctors recommended and he agreed to undergo coronary catheterization, which showed disease in two of his coronary arteries. Their openings were significantly narrowed, and the doctors feared that further narrowing would seriously damage the heart muscle itself and precipitate a significant myocardial infarction, or heart attack. The doctors explained to John that for many people, between 30 and 60 percent, a sudden heart attack occurs with no prior warning—no chest pains, no prior signals that a problem exists. They told him that one out of four people having heart attacks doesn't even have typical pain during the attack. Most important, they told John that of all the patients who "drop dead"—that is, have a sudden cardiac death—fully half of them had no prior warning of any problem whatsoever.[1] Then they recommended an operation that was performed more than two hundred thousand times in 1986 at a cost of between $25,000 and $50,000 per operation—a total cost nationwide of more than five billion dollars.

What they didn't tell him, and what they should have told him, was that there is increasing evidence that this major surgery *does not prolong life.* The National Institute of Health Coronary Artery Surgery Study concluded that "there are no significant differences among survival rates between patients treated medically and those who underwent surgery." A Veterans Administration study reached the same conclusion. Overall, those who have had surgery live no longer than those who have not.

There is a debate raging in medicine today about when this major surgery should be performed. If John Henderson had taken charge, he would have known about the controversy and might, just might, have spent his Monday morning on the tennis court instead of the operating table.

There are many aspects to this debate: When is the surgery appropriate? Who should perform it? How can quality be assured and maintained?

The technique was first developed in the 1960s. Its use exploded in the 1970s and '80s. In one ten-year period, the nation went from 57,000 operations a year to more than 200,000. The technique existed. The logic behind it was impeccable: Take out the diseased vessel, put in a healthy substitute, and surely the patient would live longer. Of course, in medicine you can't find out whether what seems obvious is in fact true until years later—when enough people have been operated on, and have lived long enough to compare how they do with those who don't have the new surgical technique. And in this case what seemed obvious turned out not to be true. The surgery does many things, and is worthwhile and necessary in many circumstances, but it does not, on the whole, let you live longer. But this kind of news—that what we thought was so simply isn't so—comes late and is not easily accepted by physicians who have already developed a "style of practice" based on the initial assumptions. According to the statistics for 1986, about 25,000 of the 200,000 bypass surgeries were performed on patients who could have been treated medically.

In a study reported in September 1987 in the *Journal of the American Medical Association,* five Harvard physicians followed 88 patients who were recommended for bypass surgery. According to Dr. Thomas Graboys and colleagues, 74 of these patients with coronary artery disease were urged by second opinions to delay the surgery and instead to undergo an "aggressive" program of medication, regular exercise, and stress management. Sixty followed the advice. In the 28 months that followed, only two of the 60 had heart attacks, neither fatal. In the other group of 14 patients who chose the bypass surgery, there were actually twice as many—four—nonfatal heart attacks. The patients who chose, on the basis of expert second opinion, to substitute a medical approach for the surgery were able to control the danger of heart attacks, avoid the pain of angina, and lead relatively normal lives.[2]

Despite this evidence, the practice continues. Almost certainly, over time, proper norms will be approached. In the meantime, the care you get may fall into the gap between what is known and should be practiced, and what is actually practiced— on you! Only taking charge can help you avoid unnecessary, inappropriate, perhaps life-threatening surgery.

Life-threatening? You bet. In 1984 alone, more than three thousand Medicare patients died during or soon after their cardiac bypass surgery—one out of every twenty patients.

Life-threatening? Yes. Life-saving? Usually not. Then does this surgery have a place? Yes, definitely, but not as wide a place as it has enjoyed. Coronary bypass surgery is unquestionably effective in relieving angina, or chest pain, and thus in improving the quality of life. The debate, therefore, is not whether it has a place, but rather what the appropriate place is.

While the debate rages, operations continue. Whether or not you have this particular surgery may depend on which side of the debate your doctor is on. Whether or not you survive the surgery will depend, to a very significant degree, on who your surgeon is and where he practices. That is because the variation in death rates from hospital to hospital and from surgeon to surgeon is dramatic. By some estimates, more than one thousand Americans die unnecessarily each year from this surgery. Whether you become one of those thousand people may well depend on where you go for the operation.

The startling variations in coronary bypass surgical death rates for Medicare were pointed out in a comprehensive series of articles by Thomas Moore and Michael York of the *Lexington Herald-Leader* in September 1986. For example, in 1984 in South Bend, Indiana, the Memorial Hospital team operated on 119 cases, and 27 of those patients died—a death rate of 22.7 percent. At the same time, eighty miles away in Fort Wayne, Indiana, the Lutheran Hospital team operated on 78 patients and only one died—a death rate of 1.3 percent.

A 22 percent versus a 1.3 percent chance of dying from the operation. Similar cases. Similar part of the country. What did Memorial Hospital do? They replaced their surgeons, and the death rate dropped to 3.7 percent, a figure below the national average.

The following chart is taken from the *Herald-Leader* newspaper series and shows the highest and the lowest death rates for coronary bypass surgery among Medicare patients.

HOSPITALS WITH HIGHEST, LOWEST BYPASS DEATH RATES
HIGHEST

Here are 10 hospitals that federal records show as having had the highest death rates for coronary bypass surgery on Medicare patients, among the 494 hospitals reporting that they performed 30 or more operations in 1984.

State	City	Hospital	Cases	Deaths	Rate
Indiana	South Bend	Memorial Hospital	119	27	22.7
Illinois	Chicago	Michael Reese Hospital Medical Center	40	8	20.0
Pennsylvania	Philadelphia	Hospital of the Medical College of Pa.	50	10	20.0
Nevada	Las Vegas	Humana Hospital Sunrise	81	16	19.8
Colorado	Colorado Springs	Memorial Hospital	51	9	17.6
California	San Francisco	Pacific Presbyterian Hospital	86	15	17.4
	Monterey Park	Garfield Medical Center	47	8	17.0
Michigan	Detroit	Henry Ford Hospital	65	11	16.9
	Petoskey	Northern Michigan Hospital	54	9	16.7
	Muskegon	Mercy Hospital	31	5	16.1

HOSPITALS WITH HIGHEST, LOWEST BYPASS DEATH RATES
LOWEST

Federal records showed 107 hospitals achieved a mortality rate of 3 percent or less on coronary bypass operations on Medicare patients in 1984, a rate that experts said was excellent. Only hospitals performing 30 or more operations were included. Here are hospitals in surrounding states in that group.

State	City	Hospital	Cases	Deaths	Rate
Illinois	Maywood	Foster G. McGaw Hospital	388	7	1.8
	Oak Lawn	Christ Hospital	94	2	2.1
	Rockford	Rockford Memorial Hospital	49	0	0.0
	Urbana	Mercy Hospital	57	0	0.0
Indiana	Fort Wayne	Parkview Memorial Hospital	63	1	1.6
	Fort Wayne	St. Joseph's Hospital of Fort Wayne	55	1	1.8
	Fort Wayne	Lutheran Hospital of Fort Wayne	78	1	1.3
	Muncie	Ball Memorial Hospital Association Inc.	38	0	0.0
Missouri	St. Louis	Jewish Hospital of St. Louis	257	4	1.6
	Springfield	St. John's Regional Health Center	235	7	3.0
Ohio	Canton	Aultman Hospital	70	1	1.4
	Columbus	Ohio State University Hospital	69	2	2.9
	Lakewood	Lakewood Hospital	38	1	2.6
	Toledo	St. Vincent's Hospital & Medical Center	79	1	1.3
	Toledo	Toledo Hospital	63	1	1.6
Tennessee	Chattanooga	Memorial Hospital	46	0	0.0
	Jackson	Jackson-Madison County General Hospital	106	3	2.8
	Kingsport	Holston Valley Hospital Medical Center	66	0	0.0
	Knoxville	East Tennessee Baptist Hospital	107	3	2.8
	Memphis	St. Francis Hospital	51	1	2.0
Virginia	Richmond	Chippenham Hospital	80	0	0.0
	Richmond	Henricos Doctors' Hospital	68	1	1.5
	Roanoke	Roanoke Memorial Hospital	74	2	2.7
W. Virginia	Huntington	St. Mary's Hospital	46	1	2.2

Source: Federal Health Care Financing Administration: reprinted from the *Lexington* (Kentucky) *Herald-Leader.*

These figures tell you the chances of your dying in or as a result of surgery in different institutions. They do *not* tell you how much of the surgery was for appropriate reasons and how much was unnecessary. Taking charge here is a two-step process. The first is to have an appropriate indication for the surgery; the second is to find a competent place to have it performed.

How can such a life-and-death variation in quality exist? Statistically, it is increasingly clear that to be good at coronary bypass surgery you have to do a lot of it. The surgery requires a talented operating team, and their skills require repeated use to stay efficient. Though it is not always the case, in general the more you do, the better you are at it. The *Herald-Leader* found in its review that 153 hospitals did fewer than thirty operations a year, too few to be statistically evaluated individually. But taken as a group, the death rate at these hospitals was 60 percent higher than the national average. Is thirty the right cutoff number? No. Some groups feel the surgery should be barred unless a hospital performs more than 150 of these operations a year. Dr. Michael DeBakey, the most famous heart surgeon of all, would put that figure at five hundred. His hospital does close to five thousand.

General rules of this kind are resisted in medicine because what is generally true is not a predictor of a specific capability. Some of the best results are achieved by surgeons who operate infrequently.

But there are other reasons that the frequency standard is ignored, and the biggest one is money. These operations are profitable, very profitable, for the doctors and the hospital. According to Dr. Ralph W. Schaffarzick, medical director of California Blue Shield, quoted in the *Herald-Leader* articles: "My own personal persuasion is that there are excessive numbers of CABG (coronary artery bypass grafts) performed and this has frankly nagged at me for the last 15 years. . . . In a cynical view, it might be said (surgeons) were not insensitive to the effect on their incomes. But then we know of surgeons who frankly just like to operate and believe the surgery is the way to treat people with coronary artery disease."

The pressure to generate income from these operations is directly opposed to the medical facts. The evidence increasingly suggests that, based on our understanding of what the surgery can accomplish and what it can't, the amount of this surgery ought to be significantly reduced. One of the nation's leading cardiologists, Dr. Eugene Braunwald of Harvard, editorializes in the *New England Journal of Medicine:* "This operation should and increasingly will be restricted to patients in whom intensive therapy has failed or in whom improved survival after surgery has been unambiguously demonstrated, rather than as a panacea for coronary artery disease." Dr. Robert Rosati, a noted cardiologist at Duke University, tells the *Herald-Leader:* "Where do all these patients come from? What they would have us believe is we are having a severe epidemic of coronary artery disease. It seems likely that we are operating on increasingly less severe disease to get more and more numbers."

Pressure to generate dollars; medical evidence saying too many operations are being performed; a wide range in the chance of death during or as a result of surgery. Taken together, compelling proof of the need for taking charge.

When it comes to coronary bypass surgery, taking charge must start long before the choice of surgeon and hospital is made. It must start before the required diagnostic workup—a cardiac catheterization—is performed. For just as the quality of surgeon and hospital varies and produces vast differences in death rates, the quality of cardiac catheterization varies widely as well. Luft and Hunt found a "highly significant inverse relation between the in-hospital mortality rate . . . and the number of patients undergoing catheterization in a hospital."[3] The general rule doesn't apply to specific individuals, but as a guide it is valuable: The more often your doctor does this procedure, the better it is for you.

But no matter how well a doctor can do the procedure, there is an increasing question in medicine as to when he *should* do it. To do the catheterization when it is not necessary may cause more problems than can be solved. According to a major new study, reported in October 1987, patients who undergo the diagnostic cardiac catheterization may actually be twice as likely to die from complications resulting from the procedure itself as from the disease being studied![4] Dr. James E. Dalen, chancellor of the University of Massachusetts Medical School, studied 3,263 patients in sixteen Worcester, Massachusetts, hospitals. The death rate of heart attack patients hospitalized with congestive heart failure was 25 percent for those who *did not* undergo the test, but 45 percent, or nearly double, for those who *did* have the test. The numbers were similar for heart attack patients with low blood pressure: No test, 32 percent died; with catheterization, 48 percent died. Nationwide, an estimated ten to fifteen thousand patients may die each year from the complications of the test, from the risk of blood clots and rupturing of the blood vessels due to the introduction of the long narrow tube into the heart chambers. According to Dr. Eugene Robin of Stanford University, the test is widely overused, in part because it "gives the impression that the doctor really knows what is going on. The numbers reinforce the feeling that he is in command." And his advice to doctors, in an editorial in the October 1987 issue of *Chest,* is to stop using cardiac catheterization except in cases of severe heart failure where the diagnostic benefit can clearly be demonstrated.

In this instance, a useful procedure, a life-saving procedure when used properly, is being overused. And when it is overused, the risks may well outweigh the benefits. Cardiac catheterization has not yet found its proper niche; a general consensus has not yet developed as to when it should be used and when it should not. That consensus will emerge over time, as more studies are completed and reported. During this interval of uncertainty, different doctors will follow very different practices. For this reason, you have to be on top of the situation, taking charge, to be sure that your own treatment is optimal.

Cardiovascular surgeons are among the most skilled and most dedicated of all doctors. They perform true miracles. They repair hearts, exchange hearts, replace damaged arteries and veins with strong substitutes. They are doers. And what they do is often at the center of controversy, in part because some surgeons are more skilled than others, in part because they tend to overuse a new surgical technique until its appropriate application is found. Because the surgery is difficult, the variability in skills has profound consequences. Because the surgery is new, there is pressure to perform it before its appropriate usage is truly understood. Part of this pressure arises from the hope that the new procedure will save lives. Part of the pressure comes from how profitable it is. Part comes from competition, the need to offer what the surgeon and hospital across town offer.

What is true with coronary bypass surgery is equally true with surgery to clear clogged carotid arteries in the neck, a procedure known as carotid endarterectomy. The rationale for the surgery is to clean out these arteries before they become so clogged that a stroke may occur. A worthy objective: prophylactic surgery to prevent a potentially fatal or crippling stroke. But what are the facts about the procedure?

When a doctor places the bell side of the stethoscope against your neck, he is listening for the characteristic sound that is made when blood in the carotid arteries is propelled past an obstruction. That sound is called a bruit. When the doctor hears the bruit, it is because the arteries are becoming blocked. Patients with this condition may be suffering from symptoms caused by the decreased blood flow—temporary loss of speech or vision, fainting, disorientation, numbness. Other patients may have no symptoms at all, and their condition is detected only upon routine physical examination. In fact, 4 percent of all Americans over age forty have neck bruits but no symptoms whatsoever. Whether or not you have symptoms, a neck bruit indicates some degree of blockage in your carotid arteries. So prophylactic surgery is in order, right? Wrong.

The operation was performed on more than one hundred thousand Americans last year. We now know that in many of them the risk of the surgery outweighed the risk of suffering a stroke. In other words, for certain categories of patients, the operation may actually kill more people than it saves. According to Louis Caplan, writing an editorial on this subject in the October 1986 *New England Journal of Medicine*, "The risk of a disabling stroke that is unheralded by a transient ischemic attack is very low, probably less than 2%—a rate clearly below the risk of serious morbidity from carotid endarterectomy."[5] In fact, according to Dr. Mark Dypen of Indiana University, around 3 percent of these operations result in the death of the patient and five times that number of patients suffer strokes caused by the surgery.

Doctors Chambers and Norris, also writing in the October 2, 1986, *New England Journal of Medicine*, conclude: "We see no justification at present for carotid endarterectomy in patients who remain asymptomatic."[6] No justification. But whether or not an unjustified operation is performed on you depends on your taking charge.

After reviewing thousands of Medicare cases over five years since 1981, in the largest study of its kind, the Rand Corporation found that 32.4 percent of carotid endarterectomies performed across the country were inappropriate, and in an additional 32.3 percent of cases, the indications for the procedure were "equivocal." "This is the first study which has attempted to measure appropriateness in a medically detailed, scientific way and found this level of inappropriateness," Dr. Mark Chassin, leader of the research group, said in an interview with the *Los Angeles Times*. The procedure is judged appropriate if its "expected health benefits," including increased life expectancy and pain relief, exceeded its "expected negative consequences," including death, infection, and a worsened condition by a "sufficiently wide margin."

There is a place for carotid endarterectomy, but it is also performed when it needn't be—in fact, when it shouldn't be. This is another example of a surgical procedure whose proper place becomes known only after it has been exceeded in actual practice. It highlights the gap between what is scientifically known and what is actually being practiced in different parts of the country. Patterns of practice have developed, and they change slowly in spite of recent evidence.

In the case of coronary bypass surgery, change may be hastened by the development of an even newer technology, coronary angioplasty, in which a catheter is threaded from an accessible peripheral blood vessel in your arm, for example, right to the point of blockage in the coronary artery. A small balloon at the tip of the catheter is inflated, and much like your home Roto-Rooter service, the blockage is "reamed out." Some clots and blockages can even be dissolved by new drugs. If coronary arteries can be effectively cleaned without major surgery, obviously the number of bypass operations will fall dramatically.

But this technology is very new. If history is our guide, then its promise will exceed its performance, and it will be overused before it is appropriately used. Already it seems that the blockages recur after coronary angioplasty, just as they sometimes do after surgery. Coronary angioplasty is not a suitable replacement for surgery in many circumstances. But it is in some. Taking charge requires that you ask about and evaluate the applicability of this new technology in your case.

Controversy in cardiovascular medicine is not limited to surgical procedures. Traditional therapies are also being reexamined, and the hottest controversy now surrounds the commonest problem—the treatment of high blood pressure, hypertension.

Sixty million Americans have some degree of high blood pressure. The costs of treating this disease exceeded eight billion dollars last year alone, and newer, more expensive drugs are now being marketed. The costs of treatment are going up and will continue to do so. But if you have high blood pressure, what should you know about the benefits of treatment? You should know this: For certain degrees of high blood pressure, the treatments may make things worse—and certainly won't make things better! Remember: hypertension is a chronic disease. Once you start taking a medication, the chances are you will continue taking it for as long as you live. In such a circumstance, you want to be sure the medicine is helping, not hurting the situation.

High blood pressure increases your chances of a cardiovascular accident—a stroke or an aneurysm—and it increases your risk of developing coronary artery disease. The higher the blood pressure, the higher the risks. This observation led to the sensible conclusion that if the blood pressure could be brought down to normal, the risks would be lowered or even disappear. A logical theory. Here are the actual results: Seventy percent of all patients who walk into a doctor's office and are diagnosed for the first time as having high blood pressure will walk out with a prescription to fill. Perhaps as many as one million people who fill those prescriptions are doing so needlessly, with little or no hope of benefit from the drug.

How can that be? Because once again what seems logical isn't so. Treating and lowering blood pressure with available drugs has no effect on preventing coronary disease. It does affect the chance of stroke and other cardiovascular accidents, but not coronary artery disease. So for all those cases where the blood pressure is only mildly to moderately elevated, and thus where the risk of stroke is small, the value of drug treatment is open to question.

Everyone agrees that marked blood pressure elevations should be treated, but the consensus breaks down on how to treat the mild cases. Scientific evidence is increasingly conclusive that the common practice of treating the mild cases is at best ineffective and at worst harmful. For example, Paul Leren and Anders Helgeland found these results in their study of 785 men with mild hypertension, reported in the *American Journal of Medicine*'s special supplement on hypertension in February 1986. "The lack of effect of antihypertensive drugs on the incidence of coronary heart disease is in contrast to their preventive effect on stroke. . . . The fact that antihypertensive drug therapy has *no* demonstrated effect on the incidence of coronary heart disease is *a major health problem* and a challenge to the medical profession." Furthermore, they suggested that "the adverse metabolic effects of commonly used antihypertensive agents *counteract* the beneficial effect ascribed to a reduction in blood pressure." Their conclusion: *"The fact that a reduction in the incidence of coronary heart disease has not been correlated with the reduction in blood pressure achieved with antihypertensive drug therapy should provoke*

immediate and widespread concern over the drugs currently used.
The benefit ascribed to a reduction in blood pressure should not
be erased by an elevation of other risk factors [emphasis added]."[7]

In the same supplement, Myron Weinberger writes in a separate analysis, "This inconsistency in demonstrating even a modest
benefit in the reduction of coronary artery disease prevalence and
mortality rate has raised concern about the sweeping recommendations for blood pressure reduction in all hypertensive patients."[8]

The fact that the drugs don't work to prevent coronary artery
disease must be combined with two other factors. They have real
side effects. They are expensive. The physical side effects can
seriously affect your quality of life, and sometimes that change is
apparent not to you, not to your doctor, but to your family. In
fact, Dr. Peter Rudd, at a Stanford School of Medicine Grand
Rounds on this subject, summarized a study of "Results of Antihypertensive Agents on Quality of Life:" Out of seventy-five
patients, 48 percent thought the drug improved the quality of
their lives, *all* their physicians thought it did, but only 1 percent
of their families saw any improvement. On the other hand, *no*
physicians thought the drug had any adverse effect, 9 percent of
the patients did, and 99 percent of the patients' relatives believed
the quality of life of their loved ones—and thus their family life
together—was worse with the medication. Of these, nineteen felt
the quality was mildly worse due to their relatives' decreased
energy, increased irritability, and hypochondria. Thirty-three felt
the quality was moderately worse, and twenty-two believed it was
dramatically worse!

What about the costs of the medication? The highest risk
groups for high blood pressure are blacks and the elderly, two
groups that, on the whole, can least afford the treatments. In fact,

some studies show that nearly 30 percent of black men and 34.1 percent of black women can't afford to fill their prescriptions.[9] The irony is that some who need the drug can't afford it and can't get it. Others who may not need it scrimp and save and sacrifice so they can buy it.

The result is that many people with mildly high blood pressure are getting drugs prescribed for them that do them no good, put them at risk of side effects, possibly decrease the quality of their family life, and put a real strain on their budget. Remember, as many as one third of all patients who have increased blood pressure on one office visit will have a normal blood pressure on subsequent visits even if nothing is done![10] People in this category obviously don't need drugs and their risks cannot be justified. Others may have permanently but mildly elevated blood pressure. Whether or not drugs are prescribed will depend more on who the doctor is than on what the patient's blood pressure is. Sometimes the doctor's decision to prescribe for a mild case is right. Often it is wrong. Taking charge will help you determine what is best in your own individual case. And that decision should be based on many factors, among them whether you smoke, have diabetes or cardiac abnormalities, etc. And it should be based on an understanding of what the goal of your treatment is, whether there is scientific evidence that the treatment can achieve it, and what the risks are.

High blood pressure is common. Diagnosis is easy. Drugs are available. They are expensive, and they definitely lower blood pressure. Taking charge will help you determine if the benefits of taking these drugs outweigh the risks—for you.

DRUGS

On a cool May morning, after years of frustration and failure, Judy Brown experienced the happiest moment she had ever known: She gave birth to a seven-pound baby girl. She had all but given up hope of ever delivering a baby. Four miscarriages in five years had nearly driven her to despair. But her doctor had one miracle up his sleeve, a new drug called DES (diethylstilbesterol), and it might, just might, prevent another miscarriage. And for Judy it did. It really was a miracle.

She did not know, indeed could not have known, that it was a Faustian miracle. The price of life paid by her daughter was a deadly disease caused by the very drug which enabled her to be born. It was a cancer which would strike her down in her youth—vaginal cancer.

We now know, because of brilliant medical detective work, that DES taken by women to prevent miscarriage in the 1950s caused vaginal cancer in their daughters twenty years later. What seemed a medical lifesaver turned, for some people, into a cruel life taker. And it was no one's fault, because no one could have known.

. . .

Cynthia Ames was thirty-five years old in 1964. She had two healthy children, a good marriage, and a full-time job. Life was good, if hectic, but her family was always short of cash. The last thing that Cynthia and her husband wanted at this time was another child; they hadn't the time or the money. Cynthia wanted to be sure she wouldn't get pregnant, at least for a while. In two or three years, if things went well financially, perhaps. But not now. So she took, under her physician's supervision, birth control pills. Eighteen months later, in the early evening, Cynthia suffered a massive pulmonary embolus from which she never recovered. This tragedy seemed unusual to her doctor; Cynthia was too young and healthy. Unknown to her doctor, other young women and their physicians were living through similar nightmares. What had seemed to the medical profession and the pharmaceutical industry to be a very low-risk, highly effective method of contraception had some devastating and unanticipated side effects that were discovered only after enough people of different ages had taken the drug over a long enough period of time.

In 1987, the medical detectives solved another mystery. The oral contraceptives that had been used back then presented unique risks to women thirty-five years and older. Among them was the risk of blood clots. It was no one's fault; no one expected it. But it caused serious illness and even death.

John Howe had never even had an upset stomach, let alone the kind of cramps and bloody diarrhea that had landed him in intensive care. He had no warning that this would happen to him. In fact, he had been on antibiotics for another seemingly unrelated infection. What neither John Howe nor his doctors knew was that the antibiotic he was taking to cure his infection was at the same time causing his colitis. The antibiotic, clindamycin, was marketed in 1970, but it wasn't until 1972 that the medical profession was warned about this side effect. It had to be used widely before the data could make clear that the drug could cause this particularly virulent form of colitis. Another antibiotic, marketed in 1965, was found years later to cause the same dread form of colitis. The Food and Drug Administration first issued its warnings in 1970.

For years, nurseries for the newborn, trying to provide a germ-free environment, scrubbed babies with hexachlorophene. This antiseptic was first marketed in the United States before 1950. It was not until 1971 that we learned how dangerous this drug is, how it actually caused the most horrifying brain damage to infants. Not, thankfully, in all cases; not even in most cases, but in enough cases to establish the cause-and-effect relationship beyond any doubt. Only after it had been in wide use, and enough damage had occurred, could medical detectives solve the mystery and the Food and Drug Administration take effective action.

In 1957, medical science exulted over the discovery of tolbutamide, a pill that diabetics could take to control their blood sugar without the need for insulin injections. It could not replace insulin for everyone, but seemed effective in mild cases. Thirteen years later, it turned out that the drug itself significantly increased the patient's chances of death from cardiovascular disease. What was thought to be useful in 1957 was known to be harmful in 1970. The doctors who prescribed it acted in good faith; the companies that made it acted in good faith. The patients who took it paid a very high price.

. . .

Isoniazid appeared on the American market in 1952 for the treatment of tuberculosis. By 1969, medical scientists learned that the drug taken to combat tuberculosis was itself the cause of hepatitis. When it came on the market, there was no suspicion that the liver would react so violently to the drug in some cases. Now there is no doubt. And no way to predict who among those who take the drug will contract the disease.

Mary Jones was a very uncomfortable forty-eight-year-old woman with hot flashes, general discomfort, mood swings. Menopause. In the 1970s, the medical profession knew just what to do for Mary Jones, and thousands and thousands of women like her. They put the women on estrogens. So much estrogen was prescribed that it became one of the most prescribed drugs in the country—until 1975, when it was shown that taking those doses of estrogen increased the risk of uterine cancer. And then use of the drug in that manner dropped. Cancer was too high a price to pay for the relief of the discomforts of menopause. The use became more appropriate—reserved for those cases where the very real benefits of the drug outweighed the very real risks. The final story on estrogen is unwritten; there are unexpected positive and negative consequences of its use. But none of them was known for many, many years after the drug was widely prescribed. Today it is prescribed with progesterone, in the belief that the risk of uterine cancer is minimized by the combination. Time will tell.

In 1955, reserpine became a very popular drug to lower blood pressure. Nearly twenty years later, in 1974, the medical community was warned that while the drug was lowering blood pressure, it was also significantly increasing the patient's risk of developing breast cancer. The association between the drug and the cancer did not become clear until reserpine was used long enough and with enough people.

In 1985, physicians wrote 1,548,412,000 prescriptions. In 1986, you and I paid almost twenty billion dollars to fill our prescriptions. Those are big numbers. And behind those numbers is a very big business that has helped to make our current life expectancy and style of life possible. The strokes and infectious diseases that struck down our grandparents in their prime are treatable or preventable today. Conditions like irregular heart rhythms and weakened heart muscle respond to modern medicines. It is no exaggeration to state that we have all been touched by and benefitted from the fruits of drug industry research and development. And we have the safest, most effective drug supply available anywhere in the world.

But there are serious problems with the way drugs are prescribed, used, and monitored in this country today. These problems are so serious that not taking charge may cost you your health, or even your life!

Consider this: Before a drug can be marketed, it must undergo years of tests, to be sure it is both safe and effective *for the purpose for which the National Food and Drug Administration is asked to approve it*. Tests must be done separately *for each purpose* for which the company seeks FDA approval. It costs the pharmaceutical company millions of dollars to satisfy the FDA that the drug is safe and will do what it is supposed to do. But once the FDA approves the drug, it is *caveat emptor*—the doctor may prescribe it for any purpose, in any dosage, for any length of time—whether approved or not, whether studied or not. Thus the regulation stops when the marketing begins. Any doctor may substitute his judgment for all the scientific evidence developed for the FDA.

How often does it happen that a drug is prescribed for a purpose that has not been approved by the FDA? Very often! Sometimes to good effect, sometimes to bad. In one family practice clinic, for example, 9.2 percent of five hundred drugs used over a three-month period were prescribed for uses not approved by the FDA. In fact, two of the drugs were prescribed *more* for the unlabeled purposes than for the labeled ones. And when the faculty and student doctors at the clinic were asked whether their prescriptions for these drugs were for the FDA-approved purpose or not, they were *wrong* 30 percent of the time. That is, *they didn't know* whether the drug was approved for that purpose or not.[1]

When the 100 most common drug uses in the country in 1978 were reviewed, 31 were for purposes *not then* approved by the FDA, and 18 of those *did not become* approved subsequently. In 13 cases, the drug was used for a secondary effect—not the primary effect that had been carefully studied prior to FDA approval.[2]

Obviously, there is a wide gap between what drugs are approved for, and what they can be used for. Behind the former are years of scientific studies and mounds of evidence. Behind the latter can be anything—or nothing.

It is an incredible anomaly. On the one hand, years of effort and millions of dollars are spent in the regulatory process before drugs get to market. On the other hand, once the drugs are actually marketed and used, regulation and monitoring end. Incredibly, no formal system of postmarketing surveillance exists to monitor how drugs are actually used by American doctors and their patients.

Postmarketing surveillance could save your life. How? By detecting serious adverse drug reactions at the earliest possible time and letting all physicians know about them. By detecting important, perhaps life-saving unexpected new uses in the earliest possible time. Every one of us could benefit from information about how drugs are actually being used by doctors and whether those uses help or harm their patients.

Postmarketing surveillance is necessary despite the extensive premarket safety and effectiveness testing currently required by the FDA. Premarket testing is necessarily of limited scope, involving only a few thousand patients. Once a drug is approved, however, it can be used by hundreds of thousands of people, and only in that volume of use can rare, but potentially serious, or even fatal problems be detected.

Under the present law, for each *new* use of a drug to be approved by the FDA, the manufacturer must undertake separate, costly, lengthy scientific studies. Often the choice is made to skip the studies and the expense and let a specific new use take hold not via FDA approval but via individual physicians listening to the medical grapevine—anecdotes, case reports, or medical journal articles.

There is a drug information gap in this country between the time when problems with drugs could be detected and when they are detected, between the time when new effective uses of drugs could become widely known and when they actually do become widely known. And your health may depend on when your drug is prescribed relative to that information gap.

Taking charge requires knowing each and every time you take a drug why it was prescribed and whether that use has FDA approval. If it doesn't, challenge your doctor to show you the evidence that makes him feel it will do what he says it will. That evidence should, at the very least, show that the expected benefits of the use outweigh the potential risks to you.

The importance of this cannot be overstated. Drugs cure illness. But they also cause illness—and death. Some of the illness is unavoidable, the risk that comes when any drug is taken. But some of it is entirely avoidable and occurs either because the physician makes a mistake in his prescribing or because the patient makes a mistake in complying.

This year in America, thousands will die from adverse drug reactions. In the 1970s, experts testifying before the United States Senate Health Subcommittee placed the number from as low as 18,000 to as high as 162,000 deaths per year. And no one knows how many of those deaths are preventable. Clearly many of them are. And they are more likely to be prevented if you are taking charge, understanding what drugs you're taking and why, and being sure that your doctor is on top of the situation.

Many problems occur because doctors are not careful enough when they prescribe to find out what other medications, both prescription and over-the-counter drugs, are being taken by their patients. Yet drugs interact with one another in various ways. They can enhance one another's potency or negate it. They can set off harmful side effects that occur only as a result of the interaction. Recently 17,000 possible interactions of prescription drugs were reviewed, and 6.3 percent of them were classified as likely to cause a significant medical risk in every exposed patient; 26.7 percent were likely to cause serious risks in most exposed patients; and 19.2 percent represented potentially serious problems depending on the individual condition of the patient.[3] Interactions are not limited to prescription drugs. Your body can't tell the difference between a prescription drug and a product sold over-the-counter without a prescription. Some of the worst interactions occur between the two. For example, aspirin should never be taken with anticoagulants (drugs that reduce clotting) because severe bleeding may result. The exposure to interactions is vast. *Each time* you take more than one drug at a time, the possibility has to be considered.

Sometimes, the doctor knows that more than one drug is being taken but is not aware of the potential interactions. Sometimes the doctor prescribes without knowing about the other medication. But *you* always know what you're taking. Taking charge requires that you ask your doctor how the different medications interact. The bottom line: Make sure your doctor knows every drug you take regularly, over-the-counter or prescribed, and the potential interactions between those drugs and the ones he is prescribing for you.

In one study of 59 patients, the doctor's medical record and the hospital's record were inaccurate more than 70 percent of the time about what drugs the patient was actually taking![4] In another study, in which the records of 200 prescriptions for each of the ten most commonly prescribed drugs were reviewed for 94 practicing physicians, 1,061 problems were identified. When educational feedback was given to half the group, prescribing practice changed 30 percent of the time as a result of the feedback. The other half received no feedback, and predictably, the prescribing practices stayed virtually the same—only 3 percent changed.[5]

Why do these problems exist at all? After all, how hard is it to determine what drugs are being taken by a patient and how they might interact with one another? Why are prescribing errors made to the degree they are? There are many reasons, but they have a common denominator: education—or rather the lack of it. The plain truth is that medical students do not spend much time learning how to prescribe drugs properly; it is one of the weakest parts of their education. Once in practice, information about drugs comes too often from the manufacturers, whose interest is in pushing their products rather than in impartially educating the physicians. A physician who needs to know a drug's limitations and problems is not likely to learn them from a drug company sales representative. And the proliferation of new drugs makes keeping up on the relevant information a very difficult challenge for the physician. Once in practice, time for education decreases. But the information to master—about diseases, new diagnostic tests and treatments, new drugs—is expanding all the time.

What does this mean to you? It means you may be started on a particular drug not because it is the best one for you, but because a drug company sales representative has left your doctor free samples to give out; or because your doctor just learned about the product from the representative and wants to try it out, to get experience with it. The pharmaceutical industry spends hundreds of millions of dollars each year to get your doctor to think of their product first whenever you need a prescription. So what you get may depend more on how successful the promotion is than on how effective the product is. Taking charge requires challenging your doctor to justify his choice of drugs, to explain the alternatives and the rationale for his decision.

Overprescribing of drugs is another major problem. Although no one knows exact figures, there is a general medical consensus that too many drugs are being prescribed too often. From time to time, groups of doctors have instituted peer review of prescribing practices; the usual result of this kind of audit has been that the number of prescriptions written falls.

There are many reasons for overprescribing. The doctor is

subject to the relentless drumbeat of industry promotional efforts designed to get their products used. The doctor wants to do *something* for you, and *you* generally want something to result from your visit to the doctor. So he writes a prescription. If he doesn't, he is often asked to, even pressured to, by you. After all, you want something done. How many of us have walked into a doctor's office with a sore throat, chills, and fever, and have walked out with a prescription for an antibiotic? Probably almost everyone. Yet the overwhelming majority of sore throats are caused by a virus, and viruses are not treatable with antibiotics. How many of us have had a throat culture before having an antibiotic prescribed for a sore throat? And then waited for the culture results before filling the prescription? Probably not too many! And yet, for a sore throat, blind prescribing is wrong. Culturing the throat and selecting the drug appropriate to treat the infection is right. But in practice, it may be done wrong more often than right. It is fair to ask your doctor why you are being asked to take a drug, what it will do for you, and how he knows that it is right for your problem. Reasonable questions, of course. But how often have you asked them of your doctor?

There is a new trend that will increase the pressure on the doctor to overprescribe. Traditionally, if a doctor writes a prescription, the pharmacist benefits. The doctor makes no money directly from the prescription. But now that tradition is changing, and a brand-new fad is beginning in American medicine: Doctors are selling drugs directly to the patient in the office. This "doctor dispensing" allows the physician to profit directly from each prescription he writes. The more he writes, the more he makes. This is hardly the way to correct overprescribing. Under this system, would you be confident that you are getting only what you need? And getting specifically what is best, as opposed to what is on the doctor's shelf? If you are taking charge, beware of drug-dispensing doctors. Be sure they can justify the prescription to you. Then, and only then, should you let them fill it!

Taking charge is essential to the proper use of prescription drugs. After all, in almost no other area of medicine is the system so irrational: Regulation is heavy prior to marketing, but lax after it. A doctor can prescribe any drug for any purpose in any dosage, and no systematic effort is made to monitor how it is actually used. The physician's information about new drugs comes too little in medical school, and too much after graduation from manufacturers whose goal is to sell rather than to educate. Overprescribing and misprescribing are much too frequent; patients often end up on far too many drugs. That more people don't die or become seriously ill as a result of such a chaotic system is a testament to the inherent safety of our drug supply.

The science that underpins the pharmaceutical industry is exploding. More and more sophisticated drugs will be loaded on top of the current inadequately understood armamentarium. The need for physicians to keep up will be greater, but they will be less able to do so. In such circumstances, taking charge makes a real difference—to be sure you take what you need, and only what you need, and in the appropriate manner.

We are not all alike, and you won't react in the same way to the same dose of medicine as someone else does. This is a very important point to understand. Most drugs come in "children's" doses which are usually related to body weight. Adult doses, however, are sold in the same dosage for every adult regardless of age or size. Logic tells you that a 6'5" man weighing 285 pounds and a 5'3" woman weighing 105 pounds would, in an ideal world, receive different doses of the same drug for the same illness. But they usually don't. As a result, one person is getting too high a dose for her weight, and the other is getting too little. Both patients may be cured, or one patient may be overdosed, with a higher chance of side effects, while the other is underdosed with a lesser chance of beneficial effect. Our drug supply is safe enough that we can get away with such imprecision—most of the time.

Size is not the only important factor. Age is equally critical. Aging changes not only how we look; it also changes how our body operates. The kidney, liver, lungs, and nervous system change with age and function differently. We are the same person, but we live in a physiologically different body. The older we are, the less likely we are to handle drugs efficiently. More often than not, the organs responsible for the breakdown and elimination of drugs just don't work as well as they did. This means that a dose of a drug appropriate for a person at age forty may no longer be appropriate at age seventy.

And yet, very few doctors routinely take age into account once people have crossed the threshold between child and adult. As a result, specialists in geriatrics are increasingly sounding the alarm about the overmedication of the nation's elderly.

Remember, the older you are, the more likely you are to be on multiple medications over long periods of time for chronic conditions. That presents a higher risk of an adverse drug reaction under any circumstances. It is particularly perilous if you are older, and if each of the drugs you are taking is at a dose uncorrected for your age!

Taking charge is especially important in the health care of senior citizens. Many of us can do it for ourselves. Many of us may need help from a loved one or family member. Overmedication of our elderly is a fact of life in America. You can help to reduce it by taking charge.

DIAGNOSTIC AND
LABORATORY TESTS

L ast year, Americans spent thirty billion dollars on medical tests: to screen them, to diagnose diseases, to monitor their conditions. Many of those tests were unnecessary. The use of laboratory tests varies almost as widely as the treatments for the diseases that show up in the tests, and once again, "style of practice" may have more to do with which tests are ordered for you than your actual medical condition! According to Bernard Tresnowki, president of Blue Cross and Blue Shield, between six and eighteen billion dollars each year are spent on "procedures which do not aid in the diagnosis or treatment of illness." In April 1987 Blue Cross and Blue Shield announced an unprecedented program to eliminate this unnecessary medical laboratory testing by establishing guidelines to monitor and evaluate physician performance.

This proposal has provoked howls of protest from the medical profession, for Blue Cross has challenged the most sacred medical cow of all: the right of the individual doctor to do whatever *in his judgment* is best for the patient, no matter how different that judgment may be from the judgment of a colleague faced with a similar case, no matter how inconsistent it may be with current scientific data.

It is out of character for Blue Cross-Blue Shield to directly challenge the medical profession, but in this case things have clearly gotten out of hand. The truth is that where medical technology has been concerned, the more we *can* do, the more we *do*. If it's available, we use it. And more and more tests are becoming available each year. Test ordering is technology-driven, instead of being guided by the needs of the patient.

Nowhere are tests more overused than in hospitals. In the twenty years between 1951 and 1971, diagnostic and therapeutic services increased 500 percent *per patient*. After reviewing this data, Lois Myers and Steven Schroeder concluded that tests were not only overused but that this overuse actually "contributes neither to quality of care nor to patient outcome, may well be detrimental to care in some cases, and certainly raises the cost of hospital care."[1] To put it another way: More is not necessarily better, but it is always more expensive!

Medical tests are not only widely overused but also vary widely in cost. After studying the test-ordering practices of thirty-three faculty members for patients from the same general population, Schroeder found that some patients could pay as much as seventeen times for their lab tests as other patients. What could make such a difference? Only which faculty members were assigned to treat them.[2] When the audits of their performance were shown to these physicians, they changed their behavior, and the costs of lab tests dropped by 29.2 percent. Here at least information changed behavior in a significant way. Instead of invoking the "right of the physician" to do what he wants, these physicians changed what they did.

According to this study, many more lab tests are ordered for patients in a university hospital than in a community hospital, and the cost of a comparable illness is much higher. The standard explanation is that university hospitals are "teaching" centers, and that students must learn about all these tests, even if the tests are ordered by trial and error. But the truth is that it is more difficult for the faculty to teach students how to get along with only what you need. It is much easier to show them how to "investigate" anything that may be relevant. In any case, it is the patient, not the student, who pays for this part of his education. If physicians were forced instead to deduct the cost of unnecessary laboratory tests from *their* bills, many fewer such tests would be done!

University physicians are clearly not unique. The ordering of medical tests varies within most institutions, within individual communities, between different communities, and between regions of the country. And some of the most dramatic differences are between physicians in different countries.

In Great Britain, for example, far fewer medical tests are used. One study compared the use of thirteen medical tests in the management of uncomplicated blood pressure in the United States and Great Britain. Depending on the test, doctors in the United States used four to forty times more tests than their British counterparts![3] Why? In discussing the reasons, the authors conclude:

"We believe . . . differences in the style of practice may be the most important. Use of technology is an integral part of American medical practice and reflects a broad cultural bias. . . . In the United States, common office laboratory tests themselves have been shown to please patients, reassure them, and in certain instances even improve their functioning. . . . The findings of this study may reflect in large part this underlying national predisposition generated by patients as well as physicians."

Translation: America is a high-tech society; tests are increasingly available; having tests makes the patient feel better, more confident that his evaluation is complete. As a result, physicians order the tests in part for the psychological lift it gives the patient.

Such bunk is the antithesis of taking charge. "Necessary" tests are those that can affect the diagnosis or treatment. If there is no possibility that a test will have impact on your doctor's decision in diagnosing or treating you, then such testing cannot be called "being thorough." It is being wasteful and needlessly costly. What should make you feel better is an accurate diagnosis and an effective treatment—not the number of tests performed on you or the length of your hospital bill. Tests should not be done to give you psychological reassurance but to give your doctor useful, scientific information. The lift should come from knowing what you have or don't have, and what can or should be done about it.

Do physicians really spend your money and take your blood just to give you a psychological lift? You bet, if you let them. Remember the differences between the British and American doctors. When twenty-seven American and eighteen British physicians were asked to explain their behavior in ordering tests for the uncomplicated high blood pressure patients, the British doctors said they ordered fewer tests because they felt many of them would not significantly alter the therapy. The American doctors placed a heavier emphasis on the need to reassure patients and to satisfy their expectations about testing as an indicator of high-quality care.[4]

Taking charge requires equating outcome with quality, not quantity. Ask your doctor whether a test is necessary, and what he would do with the information he gets from it. If that question cannot be answered, that test shouldn't be done. A test is only as valuable as the use to which the resulting information is put. Your doctor will probably be inclined to do too many tests, and reassure himself that it is for your benefit—unless you are taking charge.

It is not just a matter of economics or of "psychological reassurance." Sometimes it is a matter of medical risk. Laboratory and diagnostic tests pose two kinds of very real risks. First is the procedure itself. Some tests involve the exposure to X rays; others require taking a sample of tissue for a biopsy, a process which may involve very real hazards. Neither kind of test should ever be done unless the information provided will be meaningful enough to warrant the potential risks.

Second is the risk of an inaccurate test result. This can mislead the doctor, who may then unknowingly lead you into trouble by starting an inappropriate treatment. This is a real risk. The only thing more variable than the quality of medical care from doctor to doctor is the quality and accuracy of test results from laboratory to laboratory. Many studies document this variability. The American Medical Association itself has proposed resolutions to its members calling for standards to assure the comparability of laboratory data from place to place.

Technology has made it possible to do more and more different kinds of tests each year, in different kinds of settings. The more tests there are, the more places they can be performed, the more variability there is, and the greater the risk of misleading information.

Tests are done in hospital labs and commercial labs, in public health labs and in doctors' office labs. More and more tests are being developed which the patient can do at home. The accuracy of test results varies from group to group, within groups, and within individual laboratories from day to day. In general, hospital and commercial laboratories are more accurate and reliable than those in doctors' offices. But you are not "in general," and the variability of test results is sufficiently high in each group that questions about a test's accuracy must always be kept in mind.

Here are some examples of how serious a problem this is: In 1982, the National Centers for Disease Control reported on a "blind" testing survey of six laboratories. Identical specimens were sent to the laboratories, routinely marked as if from a doctor's office. The result? Each laboratory's performance was found to be unacceptable. In other words, all six labs flunked the test. In fact, for one of the tests, urine screening for drug levels, the percentage of *false* negative results ranged from 14 percent to 76 percent. That is, although the specimens contained a drug, the labs failed to detect it.[5]

Second example: In February 1986, the performance of hundreds of clinical microbiology laboratories was evaluated by Charles W. Griffin, III. He and his colleagues found wide variability in accuracy from lab to lab. They also found that the more tests a lab did, the more accurate its results were. In other words, the more experience, the better the results. So for bacteriology tests, those labs handling 10–80 specimens per week had an error rate of 12 percent. If they handled more than 1,200 specimens per week, the error rate was only 5 percent.

The same results were found in mycology and parasitology labs. Mycology labs that handled less than 6 specimens a week had an error rate of 15.5 percent. If the labs handled more than 80 specimens a week, the error rate was only 4 percent. For parasitology labs, those handling less than 8 specimens a week had an error rate of 15 percent. Those handling more than 61 specimens per week had an error rate of 6 percent.[6]

The message: In general, smaller microbiology labs handling fewer specimens are to be avoided if you want the most accurate result possible. This means you must ask your doctor where he's sending your specimen and whether it is a high-volume facility. If it isn't, or if your doctor doesn't know, stop the process until you're certain an appropriate laboratory has been identified.

Third example: The performance of a wide variety of tests in a doctor's office laboratory is a relatively new phenomenon, and it is potentially dangerous because there is a substantial gap between the time the practice develops and the time its quality is assessed and performance standards are put in place. During that gap, many errors can be made. Consider what happened in Idaho when physicians began doing hematology, clinical chemistry, microbiology, and urinalysis testing in their offices on an ad hoc basis. Test results varied so enormously that the state stepped in to require compliance with quality assurance guidelines and proficiency testing. As a result, laboratory performance in Idaho improved dramatically.[7] A California study showed a 50 percent to 250 percent greater variation in the results of laboratory tests performed in doctors' offices than in those done in licensed clinical laboratories. With variations like these, the doctor who needs these test results to treat his patients must exercise extreme caution.

Fourth example: Two practitioners, John M. Rathbun, M.D., and Nancy Bentz, M.T., wrote a letter to *The American Journal of Psychiatry* in September 1986, describing their frustration in trying to measure the level of an antidepressant medication in their patient's blood. Rathbun and Bentz took one sample of blood, split it into three parts, and sent each part to a different lab. They received three totally different readings of the drug level from the same blood sample: 1,142 ng/ml at one place, 632 ng/ml at another, and 1,480 ng/ml at the third. Rathbun and

Bentz confirmed what the American Psychiatric Association had previously reported: a two to twenty times greater variation in tests to measure antidepressant drugs than for other drugs. If treatment depends, as it often does, on achieving an optimal and continuing blood level of a drug, then with this kind of variability, the treatment can fail.

We can test for more things, with better quality, than we ever have before, but the fact that we *can* do more tests doesn't mean that we *should*. A test is only as valuable as the use to which the resulting information is put. The fact that the tests *can* be of better quality doesn't mean that they *will* be. The variation can be enormous and can cause your doctor to make wrong decisions.

Our system encourages too many tests. The test results contain too many errors, and the whole process is too costly. All of this is supposed to be for the patient's benefit, if not medically, at the very least, for a "psychological lift." This system calls out for taking charge. The best psychological lift of all comes from proper diagnosis and effective treatment, involving the minimum number of tests necessary to do the job.

THE CASE FOR
TAKING CHARGE

The case for taking charge boils down to this: You cannot get the best that American medicine has to offer by chance. There is simply too much variation in quality—of diagnosis, of treatment, of surgical skills, of hospital care, of prescribing practices, and utilization of laboratory services. To ignore this variability is to put your health, and perhaps your life, in jeopardy. You have to participate actively in the process by carefully selecting your doctor and hospital, by understanding and monitoring your own treatment—in other words, by taking charge.

Obviously the doctor is the key. Variations in the quality of medical care reflect variations in physician ability. How can such variable quality exist? How can out-of-date treatments continue for years after new treatments are developed? Some of it has to do with how the new information is transmitted from the laboratory, to the university-based physicians, and then around the country to the rest of the practicing doctors. Some of it has to do with the sheer volume of new information coming out all the time, which the doctor must absorb while still maintaining a full-time practice. Some of it has to do with human nature, with differences in competence and ability. Some of the variation in quality, some of the lag in dissemination of new information, is unavoidable. But not all. Consider this. If airplane pilots were tested for competence at age thirty and *never tested* again before they retired at sixty, would you fly? Of course not—and no country in the world would allow pilots to continue flying without periodically recertifying their skills in the light of developing technology. Furthermore, if a pilot is to fly a new airplane— switch from, say, a DC9 to a DC10—he or she has to be certified for that new plane.

But a physician, even one who opens your heart to replace its valves, can be licensed at age thirty and practice until any age without ever having to be recertified. Medical licenses have to be renewed—yes. But not on the basis of demonstrating knowledge or competence, only on the basis of spending a certain minimum number of hours in continuing education classes—and some states don't even require that! Continuing education is the functional equivalent of getting a college degree based on the hours seated in the lecture hall as opposed to demonstrating competence in the subject you're majoring in.

Surgeons licensed in the 1960s can operate in the 1980s and perform new procedures, using new instruments and technologies without ever formally demonstrating their competence. Physicians can practice long after physical deterioration has eroded their manual dexterity. The surgeon with arthritis can keep cutting as long as his own judgment tells him he's competent.

Shocking? Yes. What would the medical profession say? They would say that the responsibility to police the profession belongs to the profession alone, that they do it and do it well, that when skills are eroded, or when doctors are incompetent, their colleagues will know and will put a stop to it. They would say that state licensure boards can and do pull out the bad apples. They would say that hospital privileges would be immediately withdrawn from any surgeon whose lack of skill endangers patients.

That is what they would say. But the truth is that only the rottenest of the apples is thrown out. The dean of the Yale University School of Medicine, Dr. Leon Rosenberg, put it very well in a May 1987 interview in the *Yale Alumni Magazine* about the current problems in the medical profession:

> Doctors are responsible for a very major part of the fall from grace. They have tended to present themselves as too interested in their own benefit and too little interested in the welfare of society. Doctors have been too concerned about being absolutely autonomous rather than functioning in a partnership in the delivery of health care.

But to Dean Rosenberg, the most serious problem of all may be the fact that doctors *"have been unwilling to identify and discipline physicians who are incompetent, or impaired,* and by doing so have suggested to the public that the *guild of medicine* comes before the responsibility to the patient [emphasis added]."

As of December 31, 1985, there were 552,716 practicing physicians in the United States and territories.[1] In 1984, the state medical boards in six states—Alaska, Delaware, Hawaii, Idaho, Minnesota, and Vermont, as well as the District of Columbia— did not revoke a *single* medical license. In fifteen other states, only one or two licenses were revoked. You can imagine what those revocations must have been for!

In that same year, 1984, the state medical boards of Alaska and Delaware took no disciplinary action of any kind against any physician. In thirteen other states and the District of Columbia, the state medical boards took fewer than ten disciplinary actions, nine other states took between ten and twenty actions, and only twelve state boards took more than fifty disciplinary actions. To find out what happened in your state, check the following tables:[2]

States Suspending or Revoking Nine or Fewer Licenses in 1984

Alabama	Nevada
Alaska	New Hampshire
Arizona	New Mexico
Arkansas	North Dakota
Colorado	Oklahoma
Connecticut	Oregon
Delaware	Rhode Island
District of Columbia	South Carolina
Hawaii	South Dakota
Idaho	Tennessee
Kansas	Utah
Maine	Vermont
Maryland	Washington
Minnesota	West Virginia
Mississippi	Wisconsin
Montana	Wyoming
Nebraska	

States Suspending or Revoking Twenty or More Licenses in 1984

California	Louisiana
Florida	Missouri
Indiana	New Jersey

States Revoking No Medical Licenses in 1984

Alaska	Idaho
District of Columbia	Minnesota
Delaware	Vermont
Hawaii	

The message is clear. Self-policing has been inadequate. The system is clearly not going to correct itself. There is no move afoot to require recertification of competence. Without that, the system of "license for life" will continue.

When all of these elements are combined—the explosion of new knowledge on an almost daily basis, the long hours required in the practice of medicine, and the absence of a meaningful system for recertification of competence—their cumulative impact on the quality of medical care can be overwhelming.

The wonder is not that quality varies so widely, but rather that it can be so good in so many places, that we can get the best medical care available anywhere in the world—and usually find it close to home.

But not by chance. Not by playing medical roulette. We can find it only by taking charge.

SECTION TWO

OBSTACLES TO TAKING CHARGE

Now you know you should. But you're afraid you can't. A very common reaction. Somehow the mind urges you to take charge—but the gut tells you you'll blow it, you'll offend your doctor, you'll end up worse off.

All the obstacles to taking charge have two things in common: They either originate from within you or from your doctor. You have to understand them to overcome them. That's what this section is about.

THE DOCTOR

Few relationships are as unequal as that between Doctor and Patient. And that extraordinary inequality has, over many years, become an integral part of the medical care system itself. Hippocrates urged doctors to "perform [their duties] calmly and adroitly concealing most things from the patient while you are attending to him. Give necessary orders with cheerfulness and serenity, turning his attention away from what is being done to him; sometimes reprove sharply and emphatically, and sometimes comfort with solicitude and attention, revealing nothing of the patient's future or present condition."

In medieval times, Isaac Israeli counseled physicians, "Should the patient not submit to your discipline, and should his servants and members of his household not be diligent in following your command quickly, nor honor you as is proper, do not persevere in the treatment."

Things are different today, of course, but not as different as you might think. "Doctor knows best" and "the patient should not question" remain ingrained in the modern practice of medicine. As Jay Katz points out in his extraordinary book, *The Silent World of Doctor and Patient*, "Throughout the ages, physicians have consistently excluded patients from sharing with them the burdens of decision; only in recent decades have judges begun to prod doctors to be somewhat more attentive to patients' decision-making rights and needs."[1]

In Hippocrates's time, medicine was overwhelmingly an art based on a bit of science. Because there was little in the way of scientific treatment for a physician to rely on, the patient's absolute faith in the physician was thought to be a necessity.

With the accumulation of knowledge based on science, treatments began to have a rational basis, and the need for blind faith ought to have diminished markedly. Well, there is less blind faith, but there is still too much unquestioning faith. And that faith blinds us to the differences, very real and dramatic differences, between physicians. The assumption that "doctors know best" is too prevalent in our society. If you believe it, you may well believe its extension—that *all* doctors know best." And if you think about it, we often choose our physicians based on that assumption. After all, we have no way to evaluate their competence. How do you pick your doctor? You may ask a friend. But is a friend's satisfaction any measure of a physician's competence? More likely it is a measure of personality. If you need a specialist, you may ask your general physician for a recommendation. But is his advice going to be based on geographic proximity and collegiality, or on quality? Are you likely to be referred to a specialist in another city? Another state? Of course not. The tacit assumption is that all licensed doctors are alike. They can do the job. In other words, "All doctors know best." But we have seen that all doctors are not alike. For things that matter, for serious illness, the choice of physician may be more important to the outcome than the disease itself. For routine or simple problems, this may not matter as much because many of these resolve themselves or are amenable to a variety of treatments, even out-of-date or suboptimally delivered treatments.

Not only do patients too often assume that all doctors are alike, so does the medical regulatory system. Nowhere are the track records of doctors recorded and published. Nowhere are differences in performance over the years routinely monitored and made available to the public. Unless a doctor's offenses are egregious, he is left alone, shingle on the door, hospital privileges intact, open for business. When you walk though a physician's door, you don't know if he or she has been in practice one year or twenty; whether he's had trouble elsewhere and has just moved to your state; whether it's his first month back after ten years in an administrative job. When you walk though that door, all too often, you are ready to place your faith and your life in his hands. And if you like him, and if your problems are minor and easily resolved, you will probably recommend him to others. And so the system goes.

It is a good system for the doctor. It is not always good for you.

Most physicians, from very early in their training, learn to foster your dependence, to assert their authority, and to maintain the fundamental inequality of the relationship. More important, from very early in their training, they are taught to hide their own shortcomings, their uncertainties, and their inexperience.

The training of a physician in the first few years after graduation from medical school is very similar to the military's basic training—boot camp. It is a test of physical and emotional endurance. Books have been written about it, medical TV shows satirize it; but the system persists, modified in degree but not in fundamental character.

How does it work? It starts anew each summer. There is a saying among physicians—"Don't get sick in July." That is because all the new medical school graduates go on the hospital wards around July 1. There they learn by immersion. On their first day, they may assume responsibility for the care of ten to twenty hospitalized patients. Under supervision to be sure, but they are on the front line. During my internship in 1969, interns were on duty every weekday and every other night. In order to get every other weekend off, the on-call schedule alternated Monday, Wednesday, Saturday, Sunday night coverage with Tuesday, Thursday, Friday night coverage. That meant that from 8 A.M. Saturday until 7 P.M. Monday, a single intern was continuously on duty. And he kept up that grueling schedule almost every other week throughout the year. You can imagine the quality of care given on Monday afternoon by an intern who had not slept, except in snatches, since Saturday morning. Did patients suffer? You bet they did. Were they told that their doctor had been up for two days without sleep? No, of course not.

That system of senseless physical and emotional stress persisted for decades. Only now is the on-call schedule being modulated at the insistence of both the young doctors and, in some places, the politicians tired of the needless toll the system has taken on the patients.

In addition to the physical strain of the hours, and the emotional strain of having to respond to seriously ill patients in life-and-death situations in a state of total exhaustion, the "learning process" is one of continual one-upsmanship. Each morning, rounds are made on all the patients, and the young doctor is peppered with questions about each one, often in a manner designed to show him how little he knows rather than to help him learn. Often this process is carried out in front of the patient, who may be treated as deaf, dumb, and mute—a "thing" or a "case." And the most demanding of these rounds is usually conducted not by the senior university physician, but by a resident, one or two years more advanced in his training, who sometimes uses the techniques of intimidation to cover up his own insecurities about the management of all the patients under his responsibility.

Thus, this year's beleaguered, picked-on intern may become next year's tormentor, picking on his beleaguered successor. In medicine there is one adage: See one, do one, teach one. The transition from student to teacher is that quick.

Under such a system, you not only learn medicine, you learn an attitude. In part, that attitude is: I could survive that; I can survive anything. If I could handle that, treat those patients under those conditions, I could treat any patients under any conditions. It builds self-confidence, but it does not necessarily build competence. Nor does it build an approach to the patient that encourages their participation in decision making. In fact, the pressure is to master the facts about the disease, not to develop a way of constructively interacting with the patients.

One measure of how inadequate the doctor-patient relationship is can be seen in the evolution of "informed consent" as a legal requirement. Today, informed consent is an accepted principle of American medical practice, but as Jay Katz points out, the legal doctrine of informed consent is only slightly more than twenty-five years old. For years, the profession opposed it. Yet its purpose is simply to obligate physicians "to disclose and explain to the patient in language as simple as necessary the nature of the ailment, the nature of the proposed treatment, the probability of success or of alternatives, and perhaps the risks of unfortunate results and unforeseen conditions within the body."[2]

That such simple principles could be considered controversial tells how skewed the doctor-patient relationship has been, and how ingrained the physician's approach to that relationship had become. And although informed consent is accepted today, you will have very few physicians prodding their patients to take any further steps toward taking charge.

The transition from patient-as-object to patient-as-informed-partner is difficult but necessary. The best doctors make it and understand that top quality care is impossible without it. That is because they recognize that the more we learn about disease, the further science takes us, the more questions arise to be answered, and the more choices have to be made. Treatments are always changing. Uncertainty is a daily fact of life. The more complicated the illness, the more uncertain the treatment is likely to be. In such circumstances, dogmatic approaches to the patient create the expectation of certainty where there is none; of sure success when in fact probabilities are at work. But just as the intern on his rounds is under pressure to impress by knowing everything about all of his patients, so the practicing doctor may feel the pressure to prove he knows what is wrong and how to fix it when he doesn't! And in America today, if he's wrong, he's likely to get sued. The malpractice insurance crisis stretches across the country and represents the ultimate breakdown of the doctor-patient relationship.

The crisis exists for many reasons. The quality of care varies widely, in part because there is so little monitoring of what physicians do. The "doctor knows best" attitude leaves the patient with a false sense of expectation which is not met. And the extraordinary awards granted by juries to complaining patients reflect the outrage we all feel at medical horror stories. And yet, while we can think the worst of someone else's doctor, we can usually maintain complete faith in our own.

THE PATIENT

Many of the most difficult obstacles to taking charge are within you. Let's face it—when you're seriously ill, or a loved one is seriously ill, you're frightened. You may feel helpless. It's a terrible time. You want someone to help, to tell you what's wrong, to assure you it can be put right. You want someone to lift the burden. After all, you're not a doctor, so how can you be expected to sort the illness out? You *want* an authority figure; you *want* to put yourself in someone else's hands. If you have a family doctor who has made the initial diagnosis, why not leave it to him to make the referral to the specialist, or to treat the condition himself if necessary? If you don't have a doctor, why not ask a friend to get the process started?

You are not alone in these feelings. In my years as staff director of the U.S. Senate Subcommittee on Health, senators and congressmen from both parties, journalists, and other VIPs from around the country came to me expressing similar feelings. Where do I go? What do I do? These were people used to controlling every aspect of their lives. Yet they were paralyzed and helpless when confronted by serious illness. They did not know what to do, but they did reach out, knowing that they had to do something. And that is the point. As difficult as it is, taking charge begins here because, as you have seen, the choices to be made here, at the beginning, are the most important of all.

Many of these internal obstacles can be overcome when you understand what they represent and how commonly felt and natural they are. After all, you are not being asked to do things you cannot do: to become an equal scientific partner to your doctor, to master technical information about your illness, or to make the critical decisions about your care. You are being asked to choose your physician carefully, and after that choice to understand what he wants to do and why, what the potential risks and benefits are, and when other opinions should be sought. In other words, you must monitor the process.

For many people, one of the greatest obstacles to doing that is the difficulty of challenging authority. To select the right physician may mean ignoring a family doctor's recommendation. Asking for a second opinion may incur the wrath of your doctor. Questioning his treatment so that you can understand it may try his patience. It's tough enough to be sick—the last thing you want to do is challenge the person who is supposed to make you better. But if you don't, you may not get better. And you will find that if you have made your initial choice wisely, the doctor will welcome, not resent, your taking charge.

Many patients feel that if they meddle in their case, they will "screw it up." The doctor will change what he usually does in order to "stop the meddling." So often, even though you know in your heart that you can't or won't comply with what the doctor is advising, you remain silent. That can be a terrible mistake.

Many treatments fail not because their content is wrong, but because they are the wrong choice for the particular patient. They don't mesh with the realities of your life. Some people just can't take medicine four times a day; some won't disrupt their lives for in-patient chemotherapy. Often, alternatives can be devised that will work nearly as well in theory and be far better in the reality of your life.

For many people, the thought of taking charge of your own care is unimaginable when you're healthy, impossible when you're sick. You can intellectually understand the need and desirability, but it's just not something you will ever do—for yourself. If you're one of those people who want to take charge but feel you can't, it's important to have someone lined up to do it for you. And that can be done. You need an advocate, someone you trust, a friend or relative who cares about you and will take the time and make the effort to take charge on your behalf.

It is often easier to do for others what you can't do comfortably for yourself. Some of us will do wonders taking charge for friends when we can't imagine doing it in our own case. The important thing is not who does it, but that there is *somebody taking charge*.

Remember, we are not talking about creating obstacles to good care. We are talking about maximizing your chances of getting the best possible care, even if you have to travel to another town or another state to accomplish this. The geographical limitations within which we live our daily lives often artificially constrict our thought processes. In thinking of options, we seldom consider another section of the country as an appropriate resource. For routine care, such thinking isn't necessary. For serious medical problems, however, the differences between cities for a particular problem may mean the difference between life and death. We have seen that clearly in the earlier section of the book. Whether it is the chance of losing your uterus or your coronary arteries, where you go often determines your medical fate. There are diseases for which a handful of doctors in each city can make a difference. There are others where a handful of doctors in a city are to be avoided.

The era of neighborhood doctoring for all problems is over, although the last thing you want to do when you're seriously ill is to leave home and your primary support system and travel to a place where you have no one. But there are times when leaving home is the best way of assuring that you return home.

Is travel necessary most of the time to get proper treatment for serious illness? Of course not. In part it depends on your disease, in part on where you live. In any case it's the exception to the rule—but an exception that might save your life.

The greatest obstacle to taking charge is that it is necessary at the time when it is most difficult to do. The shock of a bad diagnosis, or a frightening symptom, takes a lot out of us at the very time when so much is required of us. That is why it is important to get comfortable with the concept before it has to be used. If you are going to ask somebody to act on your behalf, do it now, while all is well, much as you would line up a guardian for your children. If you will be taking charge for yourself, get familiar with the steps outlined in the third section of this book and with the concept itself. The more familiar and comfortable you are with taking charge, the more routine and normal it seems to you, the easier it will be to carry out if you ever need to.

SECTION THREE

HOW TO TAKE CHARGE

Who should be responsible for taking charge of your illness?

There are only two choices: you or someone very close to you. Remember, what you need is a highly partisan advocate who cares exclusively about your interests—not the doctor's, not the hospital's, but yours. You need someone with the time, the energy, and the commitment to get involved in all aspects of your case and to see it through to your complete recovery. Remember, a doctor looks at you as a person falling within a category of disease, with statistically predictable chances of cure. You need an advocate who looks only at you, not at statistics. Your doctor may be satisfied if you are a statistical success who lives longer than anyone could have expected. Your advocate must see you as an experience of one, with one outcome worth fighting for.

Whether you act as your own advocate is a highly personal choice, and to make this decision, you must be very honest with yourself. Can you assert yourself in a relationship with your doctor? Can you do it when you feel lousy, when you're frightened, at the very time when important choices must be made? Are you capable of doing your own homework, even when you're sick, to check out doctors and hospitals, to question treatment strategies, to evaluate alternatives, to call in consultants? Are you the kind of person who can accept the hard truth about your medical condition, absorb the emotional impact of that truth, and still make important decisions and choices affecting your treatment? Are you the kind of person who would be easily manipulated by your doctor when you're sick and accept the appearance of involvement and understanding of your treatment while sacrificing the reality of true involvement and understanding?

The truth is that people often act differently when they're sick than when they're healthy. They can become less assertive, more compliant, more dependent, more frightened, less capable of taking charge. A superb advocate for others might be incapable of taking charge for himself when sick. There is no disgrace in this. There is simply the necessity to recognize your own reality, and to prepare for taking charge accordingly.

Nor is the choice an "either/or." Sometimes the best results occur from a combination, where an advocate helps the patient get the necessary information and make the appropriate choices.

But if taking charge is not for you personally, if you know it's something you just can't handle, then you must select an advocate. When you do, remember: Your life may very well depend on whom you choose. It must be someone who has your complete confidence and trust, who cares enough about you to make the necessary time available for taking charge whenever he or she is needed. It must be someone who can intelligently and objectively persist as your advocate, getting a full understanding of your condition and your treatment alternatives. It must be someone who can deal with authority figures, who can be assertive without necessarily being combative. It must be someone who can love you and feel for you, but not be paralyzed by the emotion of the moment.

Usually you find such a person in your own family or among your closest, most intimate friends. Usually, but not necessarily. Sometimes, the best choice is someone slightly detached from your life, with the right combination of analytic capability and a concern for your well-being. Remember, it is the combination of judgment and friendship you are looking for. We all have extremely close friends or family members whom we love deeply and whose analytic judgment we suspect. Such people should not be taking charge for you.

So look to relatives, look to friends, look to neighbors, but look for the right blend of qualities: compassion, affection, commitment, and analytic capability.

Even if you intend to be taking charge of your own care, the selection of backup is important. For there are some circumstances that preclude your acting on your own behalf, when your life may hang in the balance while you lie unconscious or incapacitated. In many emergencies, action must be taken immediately, on the spot, with no chance for a surrogate to take charge. But often critical decisions can await your advocate's input, and his selection of doctor or consultant or hospital can mean the difference between your recovery or your death.

Every one of us should designate someone to take charge for us when we absolutely cannot do it for ourselves, or if we are not sure we can. You really can't predict, ahead of time, how you will function when seriously ill. Selecting an advocate in advance enables someone to step in and help if you find that, in spite of your intentions when healthy, the realities of being sick keep you from effectively taking charge for yourself.

You may opt for a combination of approaches—taking charge

yourself in some circumstances, depending on advocates in others. For example, you will select your primary physician, the one to whom you go for "regular checkups" or "routine care," when you're healthy. The selection of a surgeon when you're seriously ill may be done by an advocate.

The bottom line: There is no single way that fits everyone in all circumstances. The important thing is to consider your options carefully and make a decision. You might even carry a card in your wallet with the name, address, and phone number of the person to be called in the event that you are incapacitated.

HOW TO CHOOSE
YOUR DOCTOR

We have already seen that this is a critical choice, but the principles of selection differ for different kinds of medical problems. There is always one constant: the need to find out who's good and who isn't. And there are no performance records available for you to check.

We select doctors for different reasons: for "regular" care to monitor us when we're healthy and to diagnose and treat our ordinary ills. That's one doctor. We may need others to treat a specific serious medical problem, to operate on us, to consult with a doctor we've already identified and employed. The method of selection depends on the purpose.

CHOOSING A PRIMARY CARE PHYSICIAN

"Who's your doctor?" A common question, frequently asked of us by friends who may have just moved to our area, or who may simply have never had the need to select one. Generally the question really means: Whom do you go to when you're feeling sick, to get prescriptions or blood tests done, or to be diagnosed? To put it another way, "What's your entry point into the medical care system?" Often, we ourselves believe we know what's wrong but need a doctor not so much to confirm it as to treat it, with such things as appropriate drugs, or bandaging.

When you ask someone who his or her doctor is, you don't expect to hear the name of a cancer specialist, or an open heart surgeon, a psychiatrist, or a liver specialist. You expect to hear the name of a generalist, on the frontline of medicine, to whom you can bring a variety of relatively minor maladies to be accurately diagnosed and effectively treated. You also expect a person who can recognize when a problem is serious enough to call for backup help, in the form of specialists, surgeons, or other referrals.

Such doctors go by different names: general practitioners, internists, or family physicians. For families with children, there's another name, pediatrician. These physicians serve a common purpose: They are your best entry point into the medical care system. They are, if properly utilized, the doctors with whom you will spend the most time, who will know you and your family the best. To do their job properly, they have to see you at regular intervals, not just when you're sick. And hopefully, they are the only doctors you will ever need.

How should you choose such a physician? First, you must take stock of your own particular needs and those of your family. One of the first decisions is whether you prefer one-stop shopping. That is, do you want all of the members of your family seen by the same person, or do you prefer to have the children go to one place, and you and your spouse to another, and the grandparents to someone else?

One-stop shopping is currently provided by family physicians, a specialty which arose phoenixlike from the ashes in the mid-1970s as a reaction to the increasingly narrow focus of most medical specialties. The more highly specialized the practice, the narrower the physician's focus, the more difficult it became for any of us to pick the right doctor to go to for our general care. It was as if the doctors were telling us *what* they were willing to treat, leaving it to us to find someone willing to treat *what we had*. Family practitioners, on the other hand, are willing to look at anyone with any problem. Most of what they see, they can treat; the rest they will identify as a problem, and either refer you to the right place or help you find the right place for yourself.

Family physicians are now appropriately considered to be specialists, and they are not only accredited as such, but are in the only specialty to require recertification of competence from time to time. The alternative to a family physician is a combination of general internist for the adults and a general pediatrician for the children. Obviously, this requires the careful selection of more than one individual, but if you are willing to spend a little more time, the results can be equally satisfactory.

The bottom line: You should have a primary care physician to handle the majority of your medical needs. Whether it is a family physician or a general internist is a matter of personal preference. Sometimes the circumstances, such as the particular place you live, narrow your options, but often you can make a personal choice.

Whether you opt for a family physician or a general internist, the process of selecting the individual is the same:

1. If you have just moved to an area and are leaving behind, in your old community, a physician you liked, start by asking him

for a referral. Be sure you understand whether he's recommending someone he knows personally and has worked with, or someone recommended to him by others.

2. Ask your new neighbors and business associates for a recommendation. Understand that what they say will likely be based more on the physician's personality and style than on his medical competence. But a primary care physician's personality and values affect the quality of his interaction with you, and thus the degree of trust and confidence you can develop in him. If your neighbors and friends have developed this kind of relationship of trust and confidence with their physician, then that is an important recommendation.

Remember, we are talking here about selecting someone for a long-term interaction focused on health maintenance and relatively minor maladies, not the treatment of complex, life-threatening diseases. The more serious and complicated the problem, the less likely that it will be solved at this level.

Different doctors perform different services for you, and there are therefore different standards for selection. What you think about your primary care physician as a person is more important than what you think of your specialist's personality. For a neurosurgeon, for example, his technical, surgical competence is far more important than anything else. After all, you will be sleeping through the critical part of his work!

3. Determine how important geographic proximity is to you and see how far you are willing to narrow your options based on where you live and work.

4. Interview several doctors or groups in your area, instead of simply accepting someone else's recommendation, based on someone else's experience. During your evaluation, consider:

a) The style of practice. Is it solo or group? Do you see the same physician every time you come? If not, how large is the universe of doctors you will have to get to know? How important is it to you to have one doctor? How intolerable is it to see a different face almost every time? Some people care about such things; some don't.

b) What kind of services do they offer? Can you get full obstetrical and gynecological care there, or will an ob-gyn specialist be necessary in addition? Perhaps you'd prefer to have a separate gynecologist. What kind of laboratory services does the office use? Are they in the building? Does the doctor's office do any tests? Who does their X rays?

c) What hospitals are they affiliated with?

d) How comfortable are you with the doctors, the nurses, and the receptionists, as people? Is it a friendly environment, or would you prefer, most of the time, not to go there even when you know you should?

e) What is the fee schedule? Who processes the insurance forms, you or the doctor's staff? Do they accept federal Medicare as payment in full?

f) What are the qualifications of the physicians? Are they specialty board *certified* or are they simply "board eligible," and have either not taken or not passed the specialty board examination?

Once you have completed your evaluations, compare them. If all objective things—such as physicians' qualifications, hospital affiliation, quality of laboratory and X-ray facilities—seem equal, then choose on the basis of your personal comfort. Which one was the easiest to talk to? Where did you feel most like a person, least like a customer? Who seemed to share your values? Who could you talk to, without embarrassment, about your most intimate medical problems?

Then go for it!

5. Reevaluate your decision after one year. Your choice of primary care physician is not necessarily forever. If it doesn't work out, change it. Even if there's no obvious problem, it's worthwhile to take stock after a year. Has the relationship turned out the way you hoped for your family? Would you, after your experience, recommend the physician to others? Or has it just been okay? Have you really not been satisfied? Do members of your family feel uncomfortable? Do you think you're not getting quality care? Are you not going to the doctor when you should because the expense is too great, because you have to wait too long, because the experience is too unpleasant or simply too much of a hassle?

If you're not sure, then it's not right—so switch.

Taking charge of the selection of a primary care physician involves placing a much heavier emphasis on the doctor's personality and style, and your degree of comfort with them, than for the selection of any other kind of physician. It's not that those attributes are not important for other physicians. It's just that other attributes become relatively more important the more specialized you get. Doctors who see only neurologic diseases had better know everything that is possible to know about those diseases. That's what you go to them for, not for health maintenance, not for colds, not for heartburn, not for urinary tract infection. You go to them for one highly specialized problem. Under the best circumstances, the condition that brought you to them is not chronic. They treat you and with luck, you will never see them again. It's a short-term deal.

At the primary care level, you're in for the long haul. Your family may be in it with you. The doctor is more like an extended family member—a friend, a confidant, someone you can rely on for many things for many years. So personality is important. You can't pick your relatives, but you can pick your friends—and your primary care doctor.

Remember one other thing: Today it's a buyer's market in health care. There are more doctors than we need, and there is increasing competition for you. Personal service is becoming more important as a way of attracting and keeping you. So find the right environment for your needs. There's a lot to choose from. Just take the time to look!

CHOOSING A SURGEON

Surgery: assault with a deadly weapon for the purpose of curing disease. We are made sicker in order to be able to get better. We give our life support over to machines controlled by our doctors. And some of us never get off the operating table; others get off with permanent, unexpected impairment. Some of us develop postoperative infections; others have to be taken back into the operating room because the first effort failed. Surgery is fraught with peril, but it is also as close as you can get on earth to real miracles. Surgery saves lives we would never believe could be saved; it repairs damage thought to be irreparable; restores function where none existed anymore.

Miraculous cures and unavoidable deaths are opposite sides of the same surgical coin. If you need surgery, you must not flip that coin; you must carefully choose your best prospect for cure and not leave your fate to chance.

There are two reasons you need a surgeon: One is to evaluate whether or not surgery is needed, and the other is to perform the surgery and oversee the postoperative recovery.

You should not be going to a surgeon for your primary care.

It is both a waste of his time and yours. He should be doing other things, and you need someone with a different set of skills and competence.

But which surgeon should you choose? This is a more critical decision than finding your primary care physician. If the latter choice proves wrong, very little damage is usually done and the problem can be corrected by switching doctors. The choice of the wrong surgeon, on the other hand, can cost you your life, your ability to function, or the needless loss of an organ. Most of the mistakes of surgery cannot be undone. So choose wisely.

1. Ask Your Primary Care Physician, if You Have One

Some surgical problems are relatively routine, others more difficult. Your primary care physician undoubtedly has a great deal of experience working with and observing the surgeons in your community. For the routine problems, you may well find an acceptable surgeon within your geographic area, although for complicated or more serious problems your search should not be so limited. If your primary care physician makes a recommendation, be sure to ask what that opinion is based upon—friendship, geographic proximity, reputation, or some independent evaluation of competence. Does he know how many cases like yours the surgeon does each year? Does he know the surgeon's track record with the operations—his mortality rate and his complications rate? If he doesn't, will he find it out for you? He can, although he may not be comfortable doing it. If he doesn't know the track record, or if he won't find it out, then his recommendation is mostly anecdotal—based on those cases he himself knows about and the general reputation of the surgeon among his peers. That may be an accurate reflection of competence; it may not. It's certainly insufficient, in and of itself, for taking charge of the decision.

Ask your primary care physician how well he knows the universe of surgeons practicing in the area. Is his experience based only on those who work at the same hospital as he does? Or only on those to whom he has personally referred patients? Or does he have a broader knowledge of what's going on in the community?

Remember, patterns of practice tend to be relatively constant within individual communities. Your doctor's advice may be unconsciously shaped by that pattern. You should not be limited by it.

Get two names, not one, from your primary care physician. Ask him to describe the relative strengths and weaknesses of each. This will enable you to see how candid and comprehensive his evaluation is. If he sees both his recommendations as equal and fully acceptable, and can make no effective comparisons, then there is more cause to suspect the validity of the recommendation.

Asking him to recommend two is intended to give you a glimpse into his reasoning process, and is a useful way to help you decide how to weigh the advice. The bottom line: The recommendation is only the starting point. Taking charge requires a lot more.

2. Recommendations of Other Physicians

For major surgery, it is well worth seeking the advice of other physicians. In medicine, as in every other profession, those generally recognized by their colleagues as the superstars, the very best, are widely known and agreed upon by many physicians, particularly within the apex of the American health care system, the university-based hospitals. Ask a university-based specialist for the top ten cardiovascular surgeons or cardiovascular surgical centers in the country and the same names will show up again and again, no matter who is asked the question or which university he is affiliated with. Within a given state or regional area the same kind of informal consensus exists. Part of taking charge requires tapping into that information chain. How? By calling the nearest university center, asking to speak to the relevant department chairman, and then asking for his recommendation. If you feel uncomfortable doing this, you're not effectively taking charge. It's important, so ask your primary care doctor to make the call for you. He will. Just make sure he gets all the information you need:

1. Who would be recommended if you could go anywhere, anywhere at all, to seek care. Why that person?

2. Who would be recommended if you had to stay in your own state or region of the country? Why?

3. If you live in a major metropolitan area with many top-flight medical institutions and practitioners, who would be recommended as the best person for your particular problem, and why?

4. How does the regional person compare with the national recommendation?

5. Is there anyone in your city or community he would recommend? How does that person compare with the other two?

It is often useful to call your physician's first two recommendations directly, even if you can't get to them for treatment. If it's hard to see them, ask if they have personally trained doctors in whom they have confidence and who may now be practicing in your area—or at least in the same geographic proximity.

Ask the doctors this question: If they were sick themselves, where would they decide to go for surgery, and why?

By making these calls, you will be finding out who is thought to be excellent and why, and also, how the experts themselves would weigh differences in quality of care against convenience for your particular surgical problem.

Doctors will always talk to other doctors, so if your primary care doctor will help, you will get this input. If he won't, then find another primary care doctor, because he'll be failing on one of the most important things he can do for you: helping you to find the best person at the next level of care you need; in this case, a surgeon.

You will be surprised at how many doctors will talk to patients who call them "out of the blue." If you explain why you are calling, quite often you can ask these questions yourself. The advantage of having your primary care physician do it is that he may be able to give a more detailed summary of your medical condition and thus perhaps get better advice based on it.

3. Recommendations of Friends, Neighbors, and Other Laypeople

In this area, a friend's advice has very real limitations. It is extraordinary how often patients facing a particular type of surgery encounter friends and acquaintances who have either had a similar operation or know someone who did. Having had similar surgery and survived without complications is not a qualification for judging the quality of the surgical care received. Yet there is a tendency in each of us to want to believe that we, or our loved ones, had the very best possible care. Even if we didn't. And one way to reassure ourselves that we did is to see our friends accept our advice and travel the same route, even if it is the wrong route.

Another person's successful experience is not an adequate predictor of success for your surgery, unless that person's experience is reflective of a good track record with the procedure by the surgeon in question.

Your friends can tell you some useful things. How well did the surgeon explain things? How much time did he spend answering questions before and after the surgery? Did he effectively communicate with family members immediately after completing the surgery? Was it easy to trust him, to have confidence in him? Did he take time for reassurance, for hand-holding, when needed? How did he react to requests for consultation and second opinions? Did he give a full report to the primary care physician when responsibility for the medical care returned to him? Was the operation successful? Were there any complications? Any infections? How was the postoperative care?

The weight you give a friend's advice should be influenced by one other thing: Did your friend take charge during his selection process? How thorough was he during the selection process? If he followed the taking charge approach, then he may have a lot of useful information to share with you, in addition to his impressions of the experience.

So listen to your friends. Find out what their advice is based on. Weigh its significance accordingly.

4. Check the Surgeon's Professional Qualifications

Is the surgeon specialty board certified? If he is, in what specialty? How long has he been in practice, and how stable has his practice been? Surgeons who move from community to community, from state to state, may be doing so to escape the problems that they've left behind. Are they members of a university faculty, full or part time? Do they work in a well-established group or in solo practice? Who covers for them at night?

In general, you are looking for someone board certified, who has a long and established track record with the procedure you will undergo. If a surgeon has just moved to his current practice, it is important to find out why. Most of the time the explanation is innocent enough, but every so often you will find someone who was not really moving into his new practice, but rather running away from his old one.

5. The Hospital's Record

Surgery is not a one-person show. The surgeon is the head of the surgical team, but each and every member of that team is essential to the outcome of your operation. To put it another way, any of them can kill you, no matter how good the surgeon is.

In general, good surgeons and good teams go together. But not always. The best surgeon can be undermined by an inadequate surgical team. We have already seen the dramatic variation in the hospital mortality rates *for the same operation*. In general, for complicated procedures such as open-heart surgery, a hospital needs a sufficiently high volume of cases to keep the surgical teams' skills finely honed. To put it bluntly: If they do too few, too many of their patients die.

Until very recently, the track record of a hospital was never talked about in polite company. Certainly it was not something you could easily find out. Nor did many people even think of considering it when selecting a surgeon.

Let's be clear about this: Failure to carefully consider a hospital's track record can cost you your life.

But is the track record available? You bet it is. Hospitals are beginning to use it themselves in public advertisements to try to attract your business. If there was ever any doubt about whether such information exists, just read the ads for the Eisenhower Medical Center in the *Wall Street Journal:* "If you are considering Heart Surgery, read this: Eisenhower Medical Center had the lowest mortality rate in the country."

In a *Wall Street Journal* article about the "new wave" of hospital advertising, Rhonda L. Rundle wrote: "Some marketing officials predict that health-care providers will increasingly advertise mortality and other 'outcome' figures, in part because businesses and government agencies are compiling and publishing more data on specific health care institutions. Such information, when compiled, *was kept confidential* until recently, when consumer groups began to win a long battle for disclosure [emphasis added]."[1]

Every hospital keeps records and knows, or is in a position to know, how well it does and doesn't do for particular surgical procedures. Every doctor is aware of his own track record. But until recently, that information was kept "in house," for reasons having nothing to do with your health and everything to do with their income. For who would willingly go for open-heart surgery to a surgeon known to do it poorly, or to a hospital known for an unacceptably high mortality rate or complication rate for that procedure? If you live in a community with several hospitals, and if the record of each is known for open-heart surgery, who would not try to avoid the worst and go to the the best? So the facts have generally not been voluntarily disclosed.

Until now. And the practice is changing now because of pressure from Uncle Sam who pays the bills under Medicare. The government is entitled to collect information on the claims forms about such matters as how much surgery is done at each institution and what the mortality rate is. And the government publishes this data for all to see. As we have seen in an earlier section, the data can be misleading. Surgeons to whom higher-risk patients are sent, because of their established expertise with a particular procedure, may as a consequence have a less favorable mortality and complication rate. But in general, the publication of this data has been a real service and has provided information for all of us. And the hospitals are now acknowledging that fact, by using the data themselves to get you to come to them, instead of to their competition.

So how do you get the data? Ask the hospital. If the hospital won't tell you, ask your primary care doctor to try to get it. If that fails, you can get the Medicare data that exists for that hospital. To get that, either call the Health Care Financing Administration—HCFA—in Washington, D.C., at (202/727-0735), or the nearest regional office of the Department of Health and Human Services.

The bottom line: Before you go under the knife, put the hospital's record under the microscope. If they won't tell you their track record, and if you can't find it out from the other sources, go somewhere else. If the track record is good, there should be little reluctance to discuss it. If it can't be discussed, it may be an indication of trouble ahead. It's your life. Don't risk it needlessly.

ɔ

6. The Surgeon's Record and Personality

As in the choice of any doctor, it is important to interview the surgeon before you submit yourself to him for treatment. The easiest way to find out how many similar operations a surgeon has done is to ask him. And while you're at it, ask him about his own record. I have never met a surgeon who didn't know it. You may find it difficult to ask this of the person you may decide to trust your life to. You may feel you don't want his skills to be affected by a personal dislike or resentment of you. The truth is that good surgeons, with lots of experience and an excellent track record, don't mind the questions. Poor ones, with the highest mortality and complication rates, have that record because of their skill level, not their dislike of patients. Nonetheless, your comfort level is important, and asking these questions to your potential surgeon may not be possible for you. But they must be asked, so turn to your surrogate. That's what taking charge is all about. It doesn't matter who does the asking. It does matter what the answers are.

Although personality is less important here than technical skill, it is only relatively unimportant. It's still a factor to be weighed. The recovery from surgery is aided by confidence in and comfort with your surgeon. I would never trade technical competence for bedside manner, but when you're taking charge, you're more likely to find the individual who combines the two.

If you have done your job correctly, by the time you talk to the surgeon, you will have a pretty clear idea of his reputation, his credentials, the quality of the hospital he works at, and, perhaps, what other patients have thought of him. You're coming in to close the deal, to take the last step. Whether you take it alone or have your advocate help you, it's a step that must be taken if you are to maximize your chances of making the best possible choice.

CHOOSING A MEDICAL SPECIALIST

I. For Serious Illness

Diagnosis and treatment: the two principal phases of medical care. Find out what's wrong; fix it. Easier said than done, particularly for serious illness.

The longest interval in your life may seem to be the one

between knowing you're seriously ill and finding out the cause. For that interval of time is usually filled by your imagination, by your worst fears. And yet, if you are to have the best chance to recover, it must also be filled by the work of taking charge, by the choice of the right medical specialist.

Medical specialists are the medical care system's last line of defense against serious, complicated, or life-threatening illness. They often work at the crossroads of medicine, where the incapacitation is clear but its cause is not, where the cause is clear but the treatment is not, or where the alternative treatments are clear but the right one for your particular case is not. Their job is to diagnose where others have failed, to treat where others can't.

When primary care physicians need help in diagnosis or treatment, they will refer you to medical specialists. When surgeons need help treating complications, they usually call on medical specialists. When the specialists themselves need help, they confer with their colleagues. The referral chain usually ends at a university hospital, where the most famous specialists work.

If a doctor doesn't know what's wrong, he can't treat it. If he thinks he knows but is wrong, the treatment will be incorrect. The sicker you are, the more critical a prompt and correct diagnosis becomes; and the rarer your disease, the less likely it is to be correctly diagnosed, the fewer specialists who *can* diagnose it, and the higher the stakes in finding the right person. The same is true for treatment. The more complicated your disease, the more parts of the body that are involved, the more difficult the treatment becomes and the fewer the number of physicians who can successfully carry it out.

Finding the right person is not easy. It is very different from selecting a surgeon, where technical skill may be reflected by the number of procedures they have done and the results of those procedures. You're not selecting for technical operating skills here. You're looking for a very different quality, a quality of mind and reasoning and judgment. You're looking for a medical detective who is expert in his field and can match your symptoms and test results against his knowledge of the possible diseases you may have in order to find the right fit. You're looking for someone with the skill and experience to tailor the treatment to your individual case, even if it means deviating from standard approaches. What you are looking for is called clinical judgment, a quality of mind that enables the best physicians to solve medical puzzles correctly with only a minimum number of pieces. It is a quality of mind exercised against a vast storehouse of knowledge, where the knowledge is used as a point of departure from which informed judgments are made.

Good clinical judgment can provide the margin that allows some patients to survive a disease while others don't. The disease may be the same, but the speed of diagnosis, the nature of the treatment—the skill of the physician—can mean the difference between life and death. The selection of a medical specialist in the face of such serious, life-threatening illness is often done under significant time pressure. Thus it is almost always useful to have your advocate involved with you.

How do you find the right medical specialist?

1. Evaluate the Recommendation of Your Primary Care Physician, if You Have One
If you have selected your primary care physician wisely, you have identified someone who knows when to ask for help, either in making a difficult diagnosis or in managing the treatment. If things are going as they should, he is likely to be the one who first

tells you that you have a potentially serious problem. He may not know what is wrong, or he may know but not be comfortable with treating it. Either way, he is likely to recommend a medical specialist. Most primary care physicians have specialists they work with regularly for heart, kidney, lung, nervous system, or other specialties.

The first question to ask your primary care doctor is whether the recommendation is based on his general experience with the specialist over the years or whether it is a more individualized choice, matching your particular problem with the specialist's particular expertise. Often you'll hear, "I've worked with him for years and been impressed with his ability." You need to know more. Has he worked with the specialist on this particular kind of problem? Does he work with other specialists in the same field or does he send all his problems to this one individual? If he always or almost always uses the same person, on what basis does he make that judgment? How does he evaluate the skill of others with whom he doesn't work?

Specialists, like all physicians, have strengths and weaknesses. With serious illness, the match between your problem and his strengths is important. If your primary care doctor uses only one specialist for all referrals, that match can't always be the best. With serious illness—your illness—it should be.

Ask your primary care physician whether he ever refers patients to specialists outside your geographic area. If so, why does he? What criteria does he use? Does he have an ongoing relationship with specialists in a university center, or any of its affiliated teaching hospitals? Does he distinguish between problems of diagnosis and problems of treatment when he makes referrals?

If he doesn't recommend a university-based specialist on his own, ask him whether, in his opinion, your problem is serious enough to consider traveling to a university center. If he does recommend a local university center, ask him whether your problem is specialized enough to require traveling to a different university center, because some problems are rare or specialized enough to require a treatment available only in a particular university center. Often your doctor will assume you don't want or can't afford the hassle of traveling out of your neighborhood, much less to another part of the country. Make sure he knows that for you, faced with serious illness, where you have to go is far less important than finding the right specialist. Often you will hear, "Well, if you're willing to travel, there is a person. . . ." You want to know that. At other times you will hear, "There's no need to travel. That treatment can be done expertly by the person I recommend." And for many problems that is true. But you cannot simply accept his word for it. You must take the other steps to check into it yourself.

For people without a primary care physician, the initial problems of taking charge in the face of serious illness are more difficult. Sometimes from your symptoms, it is clear what kind of specialist you need. Sometimes it is not, and without the help of a primary care doctor, patients often direct themselves to the wrong specialist and waste precious time—the time it takes to find the "wrong" specialist, then the time to find the appropriate one. If your symptoms are incapacitating, and if there is no primary care physician to turn to, the emergency room at the best hospital in your area may be a necessary first step. If the symptoms are troubling, but not disabling, your best first step is a frontline, primary care doctor. To solve a problem, you have to define it correctly. That's what the primary care doctor can help you with if he can't diagnose it himself.

When you know the nature of your problem, the kind of

specialist you need, the recommendations of your frontline physician and the reasons for them, you should move on to the next steps.

2. Recommendations of Other Physicians

The toughest diagnostic problems, the most difficult cases to treat, the rarest diseases, the greatest medical challenges usually end up at university medical centers. If your problem falls in this category, that's where you want to be. If it doesn't, you want the advice of those specialists about where to go.

University centers are primarily tertiary care centers. That is, they are twice removed from the front lines, where primary care physicians work. Doctors who work there see a different mix of patients than their colleagues in private practice. With the exception of problems they encounter in their general medical clinics, they see very little that is routine; exceptions are the only rule. University-based specialists see more serious, complicated disease in one year than their colleagues in private specialty practice may see in their whole careers. Because university specialists see more diagnostic problems, as well as more complicated treatment problems and more relatively obscure diseases, they are better able to solve the problems and treat the diseases.

All specialists start their careers at university centers where they are trained. Once in private practice, they draw their patients from the surrounding community, where there is far more that is routine and far less that is extraordinary. University centers draw their patients from cities, regions, states, and sometimes from across the country or even from other nations—from a population of very sick people with extraordinarily complex problems.

In medical school, there was a story students and interns used to tell about the difference between private practice and university practice. If private practitioners were to hear hoofbeats outside their window, they would probably think, "There's a horse outside." And 99 percent of the time, they would be right. The university specialists hearing the same hoofbeats would be more likely to think, "There's a zebra outside." And in their special environment, they would be right most of the time. When a young doctor leaves the university training program to enter private specialty practice, he'll hear hoofbeats and think zebra for the first several years. But he won't find many. And after time passes, as he watches horse after horse go by, he will gradually stop thinking zebra when he hears hoofbeats.

And that is as it should be, because there are many more common problems than obscure ones—even within particular specialty areas. There are many more treatable problems than seemingly untreatable ones. And appropriately, there are many more specialists in private practice than in university centers.

Nonetheless, when you are seriously ill, until the problem and the course of treatment are clear, prepare for the worst. Assume a zebra, and consult with a university-based specialist. That person will help you make the key decision: where you ought to be diagnosed and treated. And if somewhere else, where.

The plain truth is, when you're seriously ill, potentially fighting for your life, time is important, competence is important, and you've got to get the best help. That help is to be found in university medical centers.

How do you get to one? First, you can ask your primary care physician to make the contact for you. He may prefer that you see the neighborhood specialist he recommends and assure you that that individual will seek additional help if he can't handle it himself. And most of the time, for most of the problems, he'll be right: You'll be effectively treated locally or be referred higher up the specialty chain in time to be effectively treated. Most of the time, for most of the cases, but not all of the time, and maybe not for your case. You are, after all, an experience of one. We have seen that for serious disease, who treats you is often more important to your recovery than what disease you have. In the treatment of cancer, in particular, you run the risk of inadequate treatment if university centers are not involved. So don't take that chance. Insist on your primary care physician consulting with a university specialist. If he won't, do it yourself.

Very rarely will a primary care physician refuse to consult with a specialist at the patient's request. But you may have to give him the name and phone number of the person you want him to call. He may not know a university specialist; he may not want to spend the time finding one; he may feel you are being unreasonable. But he will almost certainly call a name and number you give him. How do you find the name? For most diseases, you can get appropriate help by dialing the nearest university medical center and asking for the department chairman for the specialty you need. If you can't get through to the chairman quickly, the office assistant will usually be able to give you the name of the right person in the department to call, if you describe your problem. If you say you need the number so that your doctor can call for a consultation, you'll rarely have any trouble. To find the telephone numbers for university medical centers, consult Appendix 3.

But just as the quality of individual practitioners varies in a community and between communities, the quality of specialty departments within academic medical centers varies within one center and between centers. And the quality may vary within a department as well. An oncology department, for example, may have an international reputation for the treatment of breast cancer, but that is of little help to you if you have colon cancer and the department does not have an expert who subspecializes in that disease. Again, most of the time, for most of the cases, the closest university will effectively perform this function for you. But if you want the best, the very best, you should take one additional step. The goal is to find an institution where your problem is one that they emphasize in research and treatment. To find that place, ask your primary care doctor where "the best place in the country is" for your problem. Have him ask the local university consultant where the center of research in this area is, where the most difficult cases are treated, whom he calls on when he needs help. You can also call on your national government: the National Institutes of Health in Bethesda, Maryland. Call the appropriate institute from the list in Appendix 1, and ask the director's office to tell you where the most research in your problem area is going on, who the experts in the field are, where they would go if they had your problem. Although government employees cannot rank a specialist's competence for you, they can, and in fact they must, tell you where they're supporting the most research in your problem area. And if your doctor calls, they will give their recommendations as to which institutions and which individuals they think are expert in the area.

I have received their recommendations countless times when inquiring on behalf of senators, congressmen, and other VIPs seeking help. If they do it for the VIPs, they should do it for you. And they will.

It doesn't necessarily mean that their recommendation is better than the initial one made by your primary care physician. But it is drawn from a much wider pool of experience, with a national perspective. And your job is to get the maximum relevant information in a short period of time in order to make your decision. With the input of the primary care doctor, the nearest university specialist, and/or the national expert you've identified, you're well on your way.

You may feel, "How can I get my doctor to call clear across the country?" Be assured. He will—if you ask him. It's done all the time. When the buttons are pushed on the phone, it won't matter to him where the ring is answered, but it may matter a great deal to you. It may even save your life.

It is only rarely that you will have a condition so unusual that you would have to travel for diagnosis or treatment to the center where a particular expert is in practice. But the chances of ending up in the right place and getting the right tests and treatment for your problem are enhanced by talking to these experts early. The important thing is to be on the right road. Consulting with university experts can help identify it for you. Often it will run through their university hospitals; at other times, it will not. But you'll be far better off for enlisting them in the process of finding the way.

3. Recommendations of Friends, Neighbors, and Other Laypeople

These are well intended, well motivated, but as in the selection of a surgeon, of very limited value. For serious illness, it would be unlikely to find friends who've had truly comparable problems. But if, for example, they have had them—such as the same kind of cancer as you—and if they've taken charge, they may be of some real help. They may have made the search for experts, identified them, and be able to put you in direct touch. Your doctor must still make the calls. Your decision may still end up different than your friend's. You must make your own evaluation.

But you might save time. Beware, however! Many people believe they've made a thorough search for the best and found that person—when they didn't and they haven't. So find out what your friends did, and how they reached their conclusion. Then make your own contacts, your own evaluation, and reach yours.

4. Professional Qualifications

There are physicians who say they are specialists and see patients in that specialty, but who have not completed the formal specialty training or become board certified in that specialty. This does not necessarily mean they are not competent. Sometimes they are not only competent but exceptional. But as a rule of thumb, a specialist without specialty board certification should raise doubts in your mind. If you can resolve the doubts, fine. If not, move on.

How can you resolve them? Find out what kind of training the specialist has had. Was he in a formal specialty training program, or did he simply take "an extra period of training" in the specialty? If he was in the formal training program, did he complete it? Did he take his specialty board examination? Did he pass?

For any specialist, no matter what the level of professional training, you should also find out which hospital his patients enter. How much time, if any, does he spend teaching at a medical school clinic? How much of his practice is devoted to the specialty? This is an essential point because, as in other areas of medicine, the more patients you see in a specialty area, the more experienced you become, and often, the better you do. Because we are training more specialists, there is increasing competition for patients. Some specialists are therefore seeing patients outside that specialty area in order to expand their practice and keep busy, just as some generalists are trying to enhance their practice by claiming expertise in a specialty area.

In general, you want to be sure that your doctor is not only well qualified academically, but in fact spends most if not all of his practice time working in his specialty. Some specialists combine their practice with their ongoing research interests. They may be fine, may in fact ensure that you're getting the most up-to-date treatment possible. Be sure, however, that the research project is not more important to the doctor than your individual care. The doctor's reputation can give you some clues. If you hear him described as a "brilliant researcher but somewhat rigid in his approach to patients"—stay away! Use him as a consultant to the specialist you eventually select.

Finally, if your doctor is new to the area, find out where he came from. If he has just come from his training program, fine. If he moved from another practice in another area, find out why.

5. Practice Setting

This is particularly important to know when you are faced with a serious, complicated illness, because university hospitals do better with the worst cases, not just because one expert is there, but because many experts are there. Many forces are brought to bear on the solution of tough problems. In the university setting, your doctor can talk things over with colleagues, call in related specialists for consultation, and order tests and X rays not always available elsewhere. The university system brings together people and technology in a setting that encourages group discussion and consultation. Conferences are held routinely to discuss a single case. It's not only an expert you want from a university hospital, but a *process* which offers the best hope of finding a solution.

Not every problem needs to be solved in such a setting, but every doctor needs to have access to a university hospital. You should ask whether the recommended specialist practices in a specialty group, in which other opinions can be easily obtained, notes can be compared, resources pooled. If the specialist is in solo practice, you need to know whether his hospital is affiliated with a university, and whether the faculty there has had experience with your kind of problem.

To put it another way: Are you getting an individual or a team? What are the potential resources that can be brought to bear on your problem? To whom does your doctor turn when he needs help?

The type of practice need not be the decisive factor, but it is important to consider when you are taking charge. You may not need more than the individual specialist you have selected, but if you do, it's important to know that the help is there, built into the process, ready to be used.

II. For Other Purposes

At the beginning of this section, we described medical specialists as the last line of defense against serious, complicated, life-threatening illness. They are, but they are other things as well. For certain parts of the body, they are not the last line, but the first line of defense against *any* illness. In essence, they deliver primary care for that organ. Some examples are ophthalmologists, obstetricians, and gynecologists. Many primary care physicians are not comfortable delivering complete service in these areas, and therefore you need an eye doctor and a gynecologist in addition to your primary care doctor.

Medical specialists are also the second line of defense for the diagnosis and treatment of difficult problems that are not serious or life-threatening. They may involve your ability to function in fundamental ways, even though they don't pose an imminent threat to your life. Diseases such as rheumatoid arthritis, diverticulitis, diabetes, Parkinson's disease, and chronic heart problems fall into this category. Some of these problems are chronic in nature, and treating them will make the medical specialist a part of your life for a very long time.

The skills you are looking for in your selection process are the same: the ability to diagnose and treat your disease. But because you may be spending considerable time with this specialist over the years—either because he's delivering "primary" specialty care or treating a chronic condition—you are looking for geographic proximity and some primary care personality factors as well.

Because the problem here is not life-threatening, there is less time pressure on the selection process. You have the time to do it right. So take it. Here's what you do:

1. Evaluate the Recommendation of Your Primary Care | |
Physician, if You Have One

Again, your primary care physician will most likely be the person who first tells you a specialist is needed, either to provide primary care to an organ system that he doesn't treat, to help him diagnose your problem, or to assist in or take over the treatment of illness. Some treatments are so specialized that better outcomes are achieved by specialists with experience. For other treatments, your primary care physician can carry out the treatment under the continuing supervision of the specialist.

Whatever the purpose, you need basic information about the referral: Why is your doctor recommending this particular person? Has he worked with other specialists in the area? How do they compare? How well does he know the universe of specialists in the area, even those not in his own hospital? Is he convinced that the problem is such that it can be handled locally? How many times, in his experience, has the person he is recommending solved the problem? How many times has he had to call in others to help? What are the specialist's strengths and weaknesses? If the referral is for primary specialty care, angina for example, where would the physician himself and the members of his own family go for such problems?

The recommendation of your primary care physician is very important for these kinds of problems because ideally, you want a specialist close to home, in your community or near it. And remember, whoever you select may have to work closely with your primary care physician, or at least keep him fully informed. So listen to what is recommended, but don't necessarily follow it until you've completed the rest of the taking charge process and fully evaluated the results.

2. Recommendations of Other Physicians

With serious illness, the presumption must always be that a university-based specialist is needed. With the problems we're now discussing, that presumption is reversed. Still, you want your primary care physician to describe your case to a university-based specialist and ask him several things: Does he agree on the nature of your problem? Does he agree that it can be competently handled outside a university setting with, or without, university-based consultation? Can it be handled in your particular community, and if so, by whom? Are there any exceptional former students of his training program in practice near you? Does he know the person recommended by your primary care physician?

Sometimes, through this process, you will get confirmation of the nature of the problem but little or no help in the selection of a specialist. You may simply be too far from the university for the staff to know the local specialist personally. Unlikely, but possible. No matter. The worse mistake would be to treat a serious problem lightly, to assume the best and be unprepared for the worst. The concurrence of the university-based specialist on the nature of the problem and the best way to approach it is worth the call in and of itself. It is, of course, best if your primary care physician makes it, because he can probably convey more technical information about your condition. But you can make the call if you prefer. It doesn't really matter *who* calls—just who answers, and what the answers are.

If the specialist disagrees with your primary care physician's characterization of the problem, or if they are both simply unsure, then the selection should be the same as for serious problems. Better to take one unnecessary trip to a university-based specialist than to end up there too late. In the unlikely event that the university specialist does not know anyone in your area, it is reasonable to call The National Institutes of Health, and ask if they can recommend either someone in your area, or another university specialist to call for such a recommendation.

3. Recommendations of Friends, Neighbors, and Other Laypeople

These are directly relevant in this instance. If your need is for primary specialty care, or to manage a chronic condition, you will be seeing a lot of whomever you select, and probably over a long period of time. So it is important to like the specialist as a person, to be able to communicate with him, to feel comfortable and confident with him—much as in the selection of your primary care physician. And here, as in that selection process, friends, neighbors, and colleagues can be of real help. Many of them have already gone through this process, made their choices, and may have had years of experience with the specialist. Ask them whom they chose and why, what their experience has been like, how easy it has been to talk to the specialist and to question him. Are things explained routinely? Does the patient feel comfortable? How many times has the specialist called in another doctor to help with the problem? What are the fees? How easy is it to get an appointment? Who is on call when the physician is off?

The answers to these questions can help you make your decision, but they are no substitute for an assessment of medical competence. And no individual patient's experience, good or bad, can be considered a measurement of a specialist's overall competence. For a patient who gets better in spite of his physician's incompetence will forever believe him to be a miracle worker. And a patient whose condition worsens in spite of his physician's appropriate, even innovative therapy, will forever have doubts about the treatment itself.

So use these recommendations for what they're worth—useful assessments of character and personality—and move on to the next steps of taking charge.

4. Professional Qualifications

The steps here are virtually the same as for all other selections. Look for specialty board certification, check the hospital affiliation, ask about the percent of practice actually devoted to the specialty, and find out when the specialist moved to the area, from where, and why.

5. Practice Setting

Remember, for most of these problems, you're selecting an office to which you'll make many visits, so it's important to know whether it is solo practice or group, and if group, how large. Will you see the person you've selected each time you come, or is it a rotating group where you may see any of the members at any visit? The style of practice may not matter to you, but if it's a group, and if your care is to be delivered randomly by all the members, then you have to check them all out. There are very different ways of practicing, so understand them and decide which makes you most comfortable. Too many people pick particular specialists only to find them largely unavailable in the group practice. That should never happen to you.

Whatever the practice, solo or group, the day of the iron man is rapidly fading in medicine; night, weekend, and vacation coverage is almost always on a pooled, rotating basis. Because illness occurs around the clock, and occasionally demands night and weekend treatment, you should find out what the coverage arrangements are. Most of the problems we're focussing on in this section are the kind that can "wait until morning." But not all. Particularly in obstetrics, you will want to know who might be there at the time of delivery. And for that type of specialty care, you have to check out all the possible hands that may "catch" your baby.

6. Site Visit to the Doctor's Office

As in the selection of a primary care physician, it is important to see the doctor's office in operation and to talk with the physician.

You're probably wondering, "How can I do that? I can't just walk in and interview a doctor. It's just not practical." Rubbish. The choice is important, to you and to the doctor. There is increasing competition for you in what is now a patient's market, particularly for community-based specialists. Some doctors may be spending part of their time in general practice and want to spend more time in their specialty.

In any event, you will not really be seeking an interview. It's more like a brief consultation. And you should be prepared to pay for the time, if necessary. After all, you may have to travel down a long road with this doctor. It is important to find out *before you start* whether you like him, are comfortable with him, can talk frankly with him. So tell him how you arrived at his office, what your problem is, and ask how he would tackle it.

How he responds to this situation—a request to talk, to learn his approach to his practice—will give you a very good idea of what it will be like to deal with him. This is of particular importance if you're selecting a gynecologist. If you're not comfortable with your choice, if you don't trust or have confidence in him, then you won't be able to confide your most intimate experiences. And if you don't, you can't get proper care.

Most people will be able to tell in a few face-to-face minutes if they can't stand the doctor. If you have that visceral reaction, pick someone else, for the relationship won't work. You'll always have doubts about what he recommends. You may defer going to him even though you know you should, and you're less apt to comply with his treatments. That's what the brief consultation is for: to maximize the chance that the relationship will work, that you will feel comfortable and be able to develop trust and confidence in your doctor.

In the long run, paying for such a consultation may be the best money you've ever spent.

CHOOSING A CONSULTANT

You have a difficult decision to make. Your doctor wants to perform a risky diagnostic procedure or carry out a controversial treatment or undertake exploratory surgery. You trust him. You trust his judgment. But it's a major decision with potentially significant consequences if it's wrong. There's a nagging doubt. You're not quite sure. What do you do?

You've been under treatment for a long time. The doctor says you're getting better, but you don't feel it. Something is not right. Is there another test to be done? What is the problem? Is it the treatment or the doctor? What do you do?

In both cases, the answer is clear: Get another opinion, a consultation.

In medicine, two heads are almost always better than one, particularly when trying to solve complex problems. The best doctors know this and welcome consultations; they usually initiate them on their own. The worst doctors resist them, resent them, seldom initiate them, and view your request as a vote of no confidence. If your doctor falls in this category, you don't need a consultant—you need a new doctor!

Many doctors fall in the middle. They know the value of consultants. They use them, sometimes fairly often. But when *they* want to, when *they* think it's necessary. Not when you do. They will agree to your request, even if they disagree, but you will know they're not very happy.

No matter. The disease you have is not under your control; the people responsible for its treatment are. And as we have seen, they may be more important to the outcome than the disease itself. So if you feel you want consultants, get them.

The tertiary care centers, the university hospitals to which the most complex problems come, have integrated consultations into the basic process of medical care. Consultations on most cases in a university hospital are routine, virtually automatic. The special advantages of such hospitals derive from having so many specialists in so many areas of expertise located in one place, constantly interacting with each other, reviewing cases together, tapping the latest knowledge available that can be brought to bear to solve your problem.

Solo practitioners, on the other hand, are on their own, not able to walk across the hall for a consultation. When they reach out, as they often do, they're most likely to call upon other private practitioners whom they happen to know.

If doctors work together in a single specialty group, like neurology or cardiology, they will probably call upon colleagues from that group for help. Multispecialty groups can offer a broader range of consulting services, but again help is usually drawn from among the members of the group.

What type of practice the consultant comes from is far less important, however, than who he is and what his experience has been. Often the reason for the consultation defines the type of person you're looking for: A complex diagnostic problem may lead a seriously ill patient to a university-based consultation because in this case you need input from several specialties. If a particular treatment decision is not complicated, the consultation may be handled in your community or even over the phone. So whom you pick to consult should depend on what you have—and the purpose for which you need the consultation.

The important point is that consultants are an essential resource for the appropriate practice of medicine, not a sign that you don't trust your doctor. It's not a big deal to use them. It's not a big deal to ask for them.

Here's when you need a consultant:

1. Before You Agree to Major Surgery

Surgery is irrevocable. Sometimes surgery is necessary; sometimes it is not. Sometimes there are medical alternatives; sometimes there are none. It is important for you to assure yourself that your

surgery is necessary and that no other equally good medical alternatives exist. Unless it's an emergency, if the surgeon says, "Let's
operate," you should reply, "Let's wait and get a second opinion."

The bottom line: You don't want surgery because of a pattern
of practice in your community. Someone with the same problem
who lives in a city with a different pattern of practice might get
well without ever coming near the knife.

Your surgeon wouldn't recommend surgery to you if he didn't
think you needed it, so the request for a second opinion will
probably have to originate with you unless your health insurance
policy requires a second opinion, as they increasingly do. In any
event, your surgeon shouldn't mind. It's better for him if you
undertake the operation with the conviction that it is the right
thing to do. Don't consult another member of the surgeon's
group. It will be harder for him to disagree with his partner, even
if he should. It's a good idea, in fact, to consult another surgeon
from a different hospital for the second opinion.

2. To Confirm Major Decisions About Tests and Treatments

The sicker you are, the more complex and unusual your problem,
the more you need sophisticated clinical judgment to manage it.
The more judgment is involved, the greater the need for consultation to discuss the alternatives and confirm the proposed courses
of action. If your problem is simple, if the diagnosis is clear and
the treatment widely accepted, the need for a consultant is minimal.

Consultants may be needed to review what your doctor wants
to do to you to make a diagnosis, or what he wants to give to you
for treatment. Some diagnostic procedures are invasive; they involve entering parts of your body to take samples or biopsies. Such
procedures may be absolutely essential, or they may be unneces-

sary, but they can involve significant risk. Try to make sure that the proposed benefit will outweigh that risk in your particular case. And if two experts agree that it will, the decision is more likely to be correct.

Some treatments are toxic—particularly chemotherapy for cancer. You get sicker because of the side effects of the drugs before you get better because of their intended effects. In this case, you want to be sure you're getting the right drug or combination of drugs in the right doses. We have seen how the quality of cancer treatment varies from place to place, from doctor to doctor. We have seen the very real lag that exists between what is being used effectively in the universities and the older regimen being ineffectively used in many communities. If you have cancer and are being treated outside a university center, insist on a university consultation—every time, without exception, even if you've followed all the steps in taking charge of the selection of your oncologist. You don't get a second chance in this battle. You've got to do it right the first time. Your doctor may be absolutely correct. Or he may not. And that's a chance you don't want to take.

The consultation can be in person, or it can be by phone. The majority of times, a phone call is sufficient. Insist that your doctor make the call to the nearest university cancer specialist, or to the nearest cancer center. And make sure that he checks the cancer center's *PDQ* information network to have the benefit of the latest information available.

The basic point is this: Treating complex diseases requires several major decisions. Think of it as several critical forks in the road. How well those decisions are made often determines how well you will recover. The more complex the disease, the more uncertainty, the less clear the treatment. Good doctors know, when they reach these points, that it helps to talk to colleagues. Maybe a colleague will have a piece of information, or suggest a test, that clarifies the choice. Consultation is not intended to substitute group management of disease for your doctor's primary responsibility, but rather to provide your doctor with the best foundation for developing specific recommendations for you, and to give you the fullest understanding of the reasons for the best recommendation when compared with all possible alternatives. With this information, you can better decide whether to accept the proposed tests or treatments. It's not management by committee; it's a support system for two individuals—the doctor with the primary responsibility for your case, and you, who must ultimately decide what will or won't be done to you.

Again, it is the nature of the problem that will define the type of consultation that is necessary, if any.

3. To Help Solve Difficult Diagnostic Problems

When doctors have trouble making a diagnosis, when they've examined, tested, and X-rayed everything they can think of and are still stumped, it's time for consultations. Almost every doctor reaching a dead end will suggest a consultant. But sometimes that dead end follows too many tests and X rays, some of which might have been avoided had the consultant been called in sooner. It is important to know, at all times, what is being done to you and why. What does the doctor hope to learn from the proposed test? What will it mean if it is positive? What will it mean if it is negative? How will the result alter his approach to your problem?

When your doctor can't find out why you're sick by the time the first set of tests is run, it's time to raise the question of consultation. Right then. It may not be the right time to have a consultation, but it's the right time to raise the question. For it forces your doctor to evaluate your status more carefully and decide whether one or two additional tests are likely to provide an answer, or whether they would be only a shot in the dark. Often your suggestion will take the pressure off him and ease a situation where he is really stumped. Other times he will assure you that he's on the right track and that the second set of tests will confirm it. They very well may. But if they don't, he's on notice, and will probably suggest bringing in a consultant at that point. The goal here is to see if your problem can be diagnosed with the minimum number of tests, X rays, and procedures. Sometimes no array of consultants can help you avoid a myriad of tests. Sometimes even the consultants will be unable to make the diagnosis. But more often they will, and the earlier they start, the better it is for you.

If the disease is very serious, life threatening, or extremely complex, involving several parts of the body, a university consultation should take place *as soon as the problem is recognized*. For less serious and complicated illnesses, there is less urgency and a much greater likelihood that the problem can be solved early, or at most, with a telephone consultation from the university specialist.

The bottom line: When you don't know what is wrong, don't give any single doctor too much time to find out before insisting that help be obtained.

4. To Evaluate How a Chronic Course of Treatment Is Going
Many problems—arthritis, colitis, high blood pressure, diabetes—are chronic. Treatments are proposed not just for days, but for months, years, even for life. Sometimes these diseases are progressive, requiring periodic reevaluation and alteration of therapy.

When you have a disease that is always with you, requiring

continuing treatment either for pain or to prevent progression, or for any other purpose, you tend to measure your progress in inches. Are you slightly better today than yesterday? Is the pain slightly more or slightly less? Do you have a little more movement in your joints or a little less? And when you measure your progress by inches day to day, you often lose sight of the overall picture. Are you better today, more functional with less pain than you were six months or a year ago? Often, significant deterioration goes unnoticed because you have gotten worse in fits and starts—two days back, one day forward, each day's movement almost imperceptible but cumulatively significant.

If you have a disease of this type, you must force yourself to shift your focus from the daily to overall trends. Measure yourself against how you were a year ago. Ask your doctor at each visit whether he can see any objective, measurable changes in the progress of the disease. Compare what he says with how you feel.

Often this process can be helped by taking stock of your condition at special times when you are more likely to remember what you did and how you felt a year ago—on birthdays, anniversaries, or holidays. It's easier for family members and friends to remember how you were on such occasions too. Often they will notice a deterioration before you do. It's important to prod them to think about the comparisons.

If the trend is clearly down, and the proposed treatment remains the same, it is time to have a fresh look—time for a consultation. It may only confirm that more of the same is the best that can be done, but it may not. A consultation may lead to something new. A fresh look, with fresh eyes, may see something new, may make your doctor aware of new treatments, new rehabilitative alternatives.

The understanding of diseases, of diagnostic tests and treatments, changes over time, even if your chronic disease doesn't.

Your doctor, seeing you at regular intervals over many years, may be out of touch with these new developments, or he may not think of applying them to you. So if things are getting worse, don't take a chance. Have someone take a second look. It can't hurt. It just might help.

5. Whenever You Want

Except in emergencies when there isn't time, it is *never* wrong to ask for a consultation. If you feel things are not going quite right, if you feel your doctor may not be doing everything he can, ask for a consultation. You may be wrong. Your doctor may have done all he could and things may be going as well as they can. No matter. Until you feel that all that can be done has been done, it is your right and your duty to get other opinions. What is simple and self-evident to your doctor may not be to you. No case is too simple for a consultation if that is what is necessary to give you peace of mind and confidence in your treatment.

Although belief in your doctor and in your treatment cannot substitute for the correct diagnosis and therapy, they can be helpful factors in speeding your recovery. Their absence can often undermine how well you do, by decreasing your cooperation with the treatment and by souring your attitude toward it. And although we don't understand why, it is increasingly clear that your attitude—good or bad—can make a difference.

The bottom line: If you want a second opinion, get one. Don't be embarrassed to ask. It's never something to be embarrassed about!

You've seen *when* to get a consultant; now we need to discuss how to select one. The process is similar in many ways to choosing a specialist.

Start by asking the doctor treating you whom he would use and why. Does he always use the same individual for this kind of problem, or does he draw from a variety of specialists? If the latter, how did he make his decision in your particular case?

Many physicians use the same consultants over and over. It can become a pattern of practice in an area for two specialists to routinely use each other as consultants. This is something you want to know, because you want your consultant to be chosen on the basis of competence, not familiarity and friendship with your doctor. You want an independent evaluation, not prepackaged confirmation. Find out the basis of your doctor's recommendation. Find out if his choice is a friend, and whether he has ever done consultations for his choice.

One of the first matters to decide is whether a university-based consultant is needed. Sometimes it is self-evident. The nature of the disease defines the type of consultation needed. Ask your doctor for his opinion. Ask him under what circumstances he would refer a patient to a university hospital for consultation. Ask him which facility he uses and why. He may say that in your case a local consultation would be fine, but if there's any doubt in your mind about that, if you feel there might be a need for a university-based specialist, then get another opinion! Have your doctor call a university consultant and ask *him* whether the university's resources are needed. And if the answer is no, ask the consultant to recommend a community specialist and get his reasons for that choice.

Remember: A telephone consultation is often all that is needed. And if you're going that route, it is foolish to be limited by geography. Once you're dialing a telephone, use the opportunity to call the best consultant you can find, anywhere in the country. To identify him, use the process described in the section on selecting medical specialists (page 146).

There are many ways to have a successful consultation. Some

require sending your medical records, and then making a phone call. Some require a visit for an independent physical examination and laboratory tests. Some consultations are best handled by conference calls among several specialists. What is best for you depends on what your problem is.

Occasionally, you will be confronted by a problem that is not serious enough to require hospitalization in a university medical center, but complicated enough and sufficiently disabling to require the best ideas of several specialists. This problem can be handled at a university on an outpatient basis. But there is another equally good alternative which I have seen work successfully many times: You can convene a conference of several specialists from your area or from any area. Each of the specialists is given the opportunity to review your case before the conference. The group then meets with you and your doctor to discuss your case and debate possible solutions. This approach is particularly useful if you are trying to review the management of a chronic disease. Because there may be four or five doctors in the room, your case gets several "new looks," all possible alternatives are debated, and whatever decision is finally reached has the benefit of all the latest information. This is a very expensive option, however, as you will have to pay for each person's time and travel expenses. So it is to be used selectively, and not everyone will be able to afford it even when they need it. But it is a way to bring the best minds in the community, or if you wish, the country, to bear on your problem.

And there are some problems that require the best minds in the country to work together if there is to be a chance for a solution. These are the problems at the frontiers of medicine, the diseases for which no known treatment exists, but for which experimental approaches are under development. I have personally seen this group consulting process save lives because of treatments literally developed in the course of the discussion itself. So if you have an extraordinary problem, you may want to try this extraordinary remedy. It's one way to assure that you get the best possible shot at getting well.

If you do not have this extraordinary kind of problem but do have one that would benefit from this process, there is a lower-cost alternative that works almost as well: the conference call. If your records are sent out in advance and reviewed before the conference call, you and your doctor can often learn all you need to know over the phone. It's harder to have a freewheeling discussion this way, but for most problems it works. And the price is a lot lower.

Whether you use a single consultant, local or university-based, or a group of consultants from one university or from several, the function is the same: to take a fresh look, to make recommendations, to consult. Not to manage. When the review is completed, when the advice is given, it is up to you and your doctor to take the next steps, to implement or reject the suggestions. Only one physician at a time can captain the team. If he is not comfortable with the consultant's approach, he won't follow it. And he shouldn't. Because if he doesn't believe in it, he probably won't carry it out very well. This is rare, but it happens. And if it happens to you, you must choose sides. Either follow your doctor and ignore the consultant, or change doctors. But how can you know who is right? If two doctors can't reach agreement, how can you decide? The answer is to get additional opinions. If the disagreement is with a community specialist, consult with a university-based doctor. If the disagreement is with a university specialist, consult with his colleagues or phone a different university center. And talk to the doctors yourself, because you want to get a personal feel for how thorough their approach is. Then decide.

WHEN TO CHANGE DOCTORS

Sometimes you will ask for a consultation when what you really want to do is change doctors, but you haven't got the nerve. Well, get the nerve. Your decision need not be forever. Even if you've followed all the steps in taking charge, you may end up in a bad situation. If you are, change it.

When should you consider changing doctors?

1. Frustrating Chronic Medical Conditions

Sometimes you need to change doctors not for what it can do for you medically as much as for what it can do for you psychologically. Some chronic conditions, such as bad backs, can drive you to distraction. They seem to go on and on, getting a little better, a little worse, a little more painful, a little less incapacitating. Bad backs are always with you. When they're not flaring up, you worry that they will. When they do, you worry that you'll never be free of pain, you'll never be normal again.

Usually these problems contain common elements: They interfere with your functioning to different degrees over very long periods of time; their cause is generally clear but the specific problem is difficult to pinpoint precisely. As a result, the treatments are imprecise, and they come in all varieties, with different doctors favoring different approaches, sometimes each with evangelical fervor.

Let's take backs as an example. A bad back is one of the commonest incapacitating afflictions. Almost everyone either has one or knows someone who does. Bad backs are also one of the hardest problems to cure because they can be caused by problems of muscles, nerves, joints, or any combination of the three. Episodes can be triggered by exercise, physical trauma, emotional tension, or just plain normal living. And these episodes can be severely incapacitating—can literally destroy your ability to work, to socialize, to make love to your spouse. They can, and they do, destroy lives. And they can linger on—and on. But most important, they can defy all attempts at treatment.

Why? Because modern medicine is often unable to precisely pinpoint the cause of back pain, and thus to intervene to combat it. Many specialties try; you could be sent to a neurosurgeon, to an orthopedic surgeon, to a neurologist, or to a rheumatologist. Each would probably treat your back differently, and the treatments would vary widely: from rest and specific exercises to anti-inflammatory drugs, or injections of cortisone and painkillers, or surgery. Sometimes one, or a combination of them, works. Often they do not. Sometimes short-term relief can be obtained, but not always.

The battle against lingering, incapacitating back pain may last not just for days or weeks, but for years. And when it does, it can have a cumulative psychological as well as physical effect on you. Even the doctors who treat you can be affected, because you are a constant reminder of their failure to effect a cure. They may psychologically give up on you, frustrated at your lack of progress and their lack of any other treatment alternatives. Some may doubt your degree of pain and incapacitation. They may feel you have a "low pain threshold." Friends may secretly wonder how your problem can possibly go on for so long. Could it be psychological and not physical? You may even begin to doubt yourself. Don't! You are most certainly not alone.

What should you do? Because the problem is difficult to solve and the proposed solutions are so varied, it is appropriate to change doctors whenever a dead end seems to have been reached with a particular approach. You may in fact end up changing several times. The purpose is threefold: to get a fresh look at the problem in the hope that a precise diagnosis may allow a precise and creative intervention; to try another treatment approach in any event; and to get a psychological boost from seeing a new doctor to whom you represent a fresh challenge and not a previous failure.

Should you change doctors every month? Of course not! Change doctors when it is clear that you've reached a dead end, no matter what the time interval.

For backs, surgery should usually be the last resort, after you've tried all the options short of surgery first. That is unless, of course, clear-cut evidence exists of a surgically correctable problem that has been confirmed by two separate surgeons. Most of the time this evidence does not exist. Then surgery can be a "cut in the dark" and should be avoided.

What is true for bad backs is true for other similarly frustrating chronic problems. Change for the sake of change? No. Change for a fresh look, a new approach, a psychological boost.

Your doctor usually won't mind at all. By the time you change, he may welcome it, having tried everything he knows or believes in, talked to everyone he can, yet failed. Remember, your doctor may give up on you because he can't think of anything else to do or doesn't believe in the other approaches he knows about. You, on the other hand, can never give up on yourself.

2. Very Serious Illness with No Known Cure
Sometimes you are faced with a deadly disease for which there is no known or approved treatment. But there are theories. There

is research. There may be experimenta!
involve great risk. The treatments may ultn.
their promise, but there is no other chance.

When faced with such a problem, as we have alreau,
must find out what is going on at the frontiers of medicin.
then go there. The question is important enough to have its ov.
section later in this book (page 203).

3. Whenever You Feel Things Aren't Going Well

You always have the right to change doctors, for any reason at all, but it should not be done frivolously. There are people who "doctor shop," changing physicians regularly for abusive reasons, such as getting prescriptions filled when they shouldn't be, or work absences excused when there is no medical reason. Fortunately, most people go to physicians for genuine medical problems. And if the relationship just isn't working out, a change is appropriate.

There is, after all, an important and delicate psychological component to your relationship with your doctor. If you don't trust him, if you come to doubt his skill or competence, if the experience with him is always negative, then it can affect your recovery. So a change is in order.

Some of you will be fully satisfied with your doctor—until you meet his consultant. And the comparison of the two may undermine your confidence. This does not happen often, but it does happen. If you feel that continuing with your first doctor would clearly be second best for you, then change. The basic question is not one of manners; you must satisfy yourself that you are getting the best care possible.

HOW TO ASK YOUR DOCTOR
THE RIGHT QUESTIONS

Selecting a physician is one thing; monitoring his care is quite another. Taking charge requires knowing at all times what is going on—what is to be done to you and why—and fully understanding what your options are. To do this, you or your advocate must be able to interact with your doctor, to press certain questions and persist until the answers are clearly understood.

Not all, but many physicians are used to controlling the flow of information to patients and their families. They want to inform but not overinform. They may want to give you the feeling of participating in decisions without the reality of true participation. They are not used to viewing patients as partners or as equals. For this reason, it is important to establish early in your relationship the kind of patient you are going to be, the kind of communication you will insist upon for yourself or for your advocate.

This should be done in a friendly way. Most of the time, if the parameters are set out early, the doctor will not only accept them but enthusiastically follow them. He should understand that you will always want to know what he finds, what he wants to do about it and why, and whether alternatives exist.

The goal is to get him to see you as a decision-making partner. To accomplish that, you must not let him do things to you without explaining them first. Remember: There is no such thing as too much information about your own condition. You may not want or need to hear everything you're told, but it is preferable to hear too much rather than too little. For if you hear less than you should, you cannot make informed decisions. If you can't handle knowing the details of your condition, then you need an advocate taking charge for you. Either way, whether you do it yourself or your advocate does it for you, the doctor has to know and accept the fact that he has a partner.

The right questions to ask depend on the situation you are in:

1. Questions to Ask at Regular Checkups by Your Primary Care Physician

Health maintenance, the effort to keep you healthy, to prevent illness, is an important component of medical care. And it is often overlooked. If you see your doctor only when you're sick, you're asking for trouble because by the time serious illness shows itself through symptoms, it is usually fairly far along. Far better to detect cancer on a regular checkup before it causes symptoms than after it has progressed to the point when they occur. Far better to detect rising blood pressure before it causes symptoms. Far better to detect diabetes early, in a routine screening exam, than after it has exacted a toll on your eyes or peripheral nerves. The examples go on and on. Serious illness can be silent for a long time, gathering strength inside your body until it explodes in obvious symptoms. Often whether you get better depends on whether you started treatment early enough.

The effort to stay out of trouble is worth your while. If you are going to make that effort, make sure that it's comprehensive. Ask your doctor about his approach to health maintenance. What does he routinely check for? Ask him, after each visit, to tell you the status of your major organ systems: heart, lungs, neurologic system, gastrointestinal tract, endocrine system, kidneys and urinary tract, reproductive organs, musculoskeletal system, eyes, ears, nose and throat, skin. He should check each one, and you can be sure he does by asking him about them all.

What tests does he routinely perform? At the very least, they should include taking your blood pressure, checking your urine, running routine blood tests including your blood lipids and cholesterol, and testing for blood in your stool.

Blood tests for cholesterol are now viewed as particularly important. In fall of 1987, the National Heart, Lung, and Blood Institute announced a new war on cholesterol, because it is now clearer than ever before that arteries clogged with cholesterol are potential cripplers and killers. In this case, you are what you eat! Almost a quarter of American adults may need low-fat diets to get their cholesterol levels down to the new recommended "desirable" level of 200 milligrams per deciliter of blood serum. If the diet fails, then and only then, drug therapy may be necessary. The government agency is calling for blood-cholesterol testing once every five years for every adult over age twenty, although at-risk patients, particularly overweight males, may need more frequent blood tests. Ask your doctor about his plans to monitor your cholesterol and other associated blood lipids. It is one of the most important components of good primary care.

You need to understand the plan for tracking your overall

health status over time. How often does he do each test and why at that interval? How often does he take X rays, and why? And each time you are checked, be sure he compares how you are today with how you were on previous visits. This is important. Ask him to explain any changes. Most of them will be insignificant, but some may be highly significant, and your problem may be detected only because of your question. For example, a blood test that was in the low-normal range two visits ago, in mid-normal range last visit, and at the high-normal limit now may indicate a significant trend. Looked at in isolation, it might be ignored, but looked at in perspective, within the context of previous tests, it might be an early warning signal. Remember, you can ask these questions only if you know the specific test results. Each time you undergo a test, you should obtain the result. This serves the additional purpose of assuring that your test result is not lost, misplaced, or inadvertently ignored by your doctor.

Finally, ask your doctor what information about yourself you should carry with you at all times. Certainly your blood type. What about your normal blood pressure range? Your blood lipids? What does he think you would need to tell another doctor who might see you when you're in a different time zone, on vacation, or on a business trip? Is there anything about you that you should be able to tell another doctor in an emergency, to keep him from misinterpreting any chronic condition that you may have as a new and acute problem?

Sometimes we go through life with funny abnormalities of no apparent medical significance. They're not normal, but they've been fully evaluated and seem to be inconsequential, at least for us. If you have such an abnormality, you should know it, so that a new doctor, in a different setting, doesn't see the "strange spot in the lung" or the "abnormal blood value" and repeat the extensive workup.

The bottom line: Know what your health maintenance plan is; know what will be checked, when, and why. And know what you need to know about yourself at all times so that you can get proper treatment in unanticipated situations.

2. Questions to Ask for the Diagnosis of a Specific Problem
"What is wrong with me?" One of the commonest questions asked of doctors. "It's nothing serious; we can treat it" is commonly all that is heard as an answer, no matter what other content was actually included. It is astonishing how little some patients can tell you about what the doctor diagnosed. It's as if they subconsciously block out the content and hear only the background music. They want to know just enough to determine whether they're in serious trouble or not.

One of the best ways of getting into serious trouble is to be unaware of the details of your problem. When something is wrong with you, you have to understand what it is. Don't accept a label for your condition unless you know what the label means. Ask your doctor what the functional impairment is, what isn't working out right. And why.

The why is very important. You want to know, if it's knowable, what caused the problem so that you can try to prevent it from happening again. Many diseases have causes we can't prevent through our own actions. But other diseases we can. Eating inadequately cooked foods, swimming in contaminated water, failing to wear shoes in certain settings, consuming too much salt or too many saturated fats, or too much caffeine, sharing glasses and silverware with others—there is an endless list of activities that can cause illness. If the illness is treated but the cause isn't understood, then there is likely to be a repetition of the behavior that caused it, and a repetition of the illness.

During my internship, there was a patient who showed up almost every night at the emergency room in heart failure. It was usually caused by his eating great quantities of very salty potato chips, which tipped his already fragile cardiovascular system out of balance. He always knew what he had—congestive heart failure—but he reappeared every night, with crumpled bags of potato chips beside him in his car. One bleary-eyed intern realized he would be awakened almost every night unless this patient clearly understood the cause of his heart failure. The intern held up the crumpled bag of potato chips in front of the patient: "These are causing your problem—stop eating these chips!" The patient agreed, but reappeared the next night in heart failure. Beside him in the car were four crumpled bags—of very salty pretzels! He had not understood that it was the salt that caused his problem.

So you have to know what your diagnosis is, and what it means, and you have to know what causes the problem—why things go wrong. And the only way to know is to ask, and to continue asking until you understand. Sometimes a problem can be caused, theoretically, by many different things, and the specific cause of your problem can't be differentiated from among them. Even so, it helps to understand what the possibilities are.

There are other questions to ask your doctor when you're sick. How will he monitor your progress? What tests will be done, and at what intervals? What does he expect to learn from these? How often will he have to see you? What laboratory facilities does he use and why? Where does he have his X rays taken, and how did he choose that facility?

In other words, you want to understand both the process and

the content of your care. If your doctor understands that from the outset, it will take far less effort to get the information you need.

A different set of questions should be asked in cases where the diagnosis is unclear. This is a very difficult situation, as we have seen, for you, and for your doctor.

You want to follow this process very closely to understand what is happening, because you may have to decide that it has gone too far with too little chance for success. That is, you may have to call for a consultant or even change doctors.

If the doctor can't tell you precisely what's wrong and why after he has examined you, ask him to outline his game plan for finding out. What tests does he want to run? What X rays does he want to take? What information does he hope to get from them? You are trying to avoid a scattershot approach; that is, when stumped, do every test, take every X ray, because something is bound to turn up. You want to be sure that your doctor has thought this through, that he has an order in which to proceed, with each step based on logic, with some promise of leading to a solution.

Some symptoms are nonspecific; they can have many causes. You will want to understand which of the many your doctor thinks is most likely in your case, and why, and which tests are best designed to confirm or refute his suspicions.

The purpose of this probing is not to show up your doctor. Some problems are very difficult and indeed are never diagnosed by anyone. Sometimes they are successfully treated by "instinct"; sometimes they are not. Sometimes they go away by themselves; sometimes they don't. So the purpose here is not to anticipate but rather to determine whether your doctor has a plan, is proceeding logically, or is confused, with no real rationale for what he proposes to do. By your questions, by your probing of his rationale, you will make it hard for him to kid himself. He will be forced to assess realistically whether he needs help, or whether he is confident enough to proceed on the basis of sound reasoning. By his answers, you will be better able to determine whether you're in good hands—or not.

3. Questions to Ask About the Treatment of a Specific Problem

It's one thing to know what's wrong. It's another to know what to do about it. Sometimes the correct treatment is obvious and universally agreed upon. Sometimes several alternative approaches are available, and it is necessary to select the best one for your particular problem. Sometimes there are no good choices. Whatever the case, you must know what your doctor is trying to do and why, and you must fully understand the treatment you will be given. For starters, you should always know exactly what your treatment is intended to do. Never swallow a pill, perform an exercise, adhere to a strict diet, or take an injection without knowing exactly how it will help you. The way to find out is to ask.

Why do you need to know? To be sure you do it right. To be sure you really need the treatment. To minimize side effects and adverse reactions that arise out of misunderstandings.

How should the process work? Let's use prescription drugs as an example: Never swallow a pill unless you know what it will do to you. Ask why you need it. See if there are alternative treatments to the product being prescribed. Ask why this particular one was chosen. Every single drug has risks associated with its use as well as benefits. You need to know the risks, the side effects, and any adverse reactions that have been caused by the drug. Ask your doctor to compare the risks with the benefits for you, the degree to which the benefits outweigh the risks. Make sure you know what to look for as a sign of impending trouble caused by a drug. Is it a headache, a stomachache, insomnia, blurred vision? If you know what the early warning signs are, you may be able to avoid more serious consequences. In other words, you should know not only how to take the drug correctly, but you should also know when to stop taking the drug because of problems.

Every time you swallow a pill, you should know whether it must be taken at meals or between them, whether it can be mixed with other common over-the-counter medications such as aspirin or antihistamines, whether it interacts with other prescription drugs you have to take. Always be sure your doctor knows every other medication you use, prescription drug or not. Why? Because failure to do so can turn a theoretically successful treatment into an actual failure in your case. How? If two drugs don't mix, they can inactivate each other, or interact with each other to make you sick. Your doctor can't warn you of the problem if he doesn't know that you take medicine for allergies or headaches or other reasons. He should routinely ask, but if he doesn't, you should make sure he knows—every time he prescribes.

It is also important to know the correct way to take a drug. The right medicine taken in the wrong way will not do the job. If a drug needs an empty stomach to be fully absorbed into your bloodstream, then taking it immediately after eating will assure a treatment failure. If you understand how a drug works, how it gets where it's going, and what it does when it gets there, you are more likely to do things correctly.

There are particular questions to ask when your doctor wants to give you an antibiotic. For many years it has been widely known that antibiotics are significantly overprescribed. One of the many consequences of this practice is the emergence of bacteria that are resistant to the antibiotics. The more the antibiotics are used, the quicker the resistance develops, and the more difficult and expensive future treatment will become. This is everyone's problem because you may get sick with one of these drug-resistant bacteria.

How can you help? By making it difficult for your doctor to give you an antibiotic when he shouldn't. To put it another way, to make it easier for him to use antibiotics as he should, and as he may, in fact, prefer to. Why is that difficult to do? Here is an example from the everyday practice of medicine: the treatment of sore throats. Fact: Antibiotics are effective against bacteria, not viruses. Fact: The overwhelming number of sore throats—more than 95 percent—are caused by viruses. Fact: Antibiotics do nothing to cure viral sore throats. Fact: You can find out whether a sore throat is caused by a bacterium or a virus by taking a throat culture, so there's no need to guess. Fact: It's almost impossible for the doctor to tell by looking at a throat whether it is a bacterial or viral problem, and it's almost impossible for the patient to tell on the basis of the severity of the pain.

So what's the problem? It seems easy. If you have a sore throat, have a throat culture taken and then treat it with antibiotics only if it's caused by a bacterium. If it is, find out what drug the bacterium is most sensitive to, and use it.

That's how it should be done. But not the way it is usually done. The truth is that many people want to take antibiotics for a sore throat; they ask the doctor for them, pressure him not to waste the visit by letting them go home empty-handed. And many doctors feel it's easier to write a prescription than to put the patient to the expense of a throat culture. They reason: If it is a virus, no harm done. If it is a bacterium, I've started the patient on a treatment without the delay of waiting for throat culture results.

Some doctors do both: They take a throat culture *and* start the patient on antibiotics. If the culture is negative, they tell the patient to stop taking the drug.

Each year, millions of tablets of antibiotics are swallowed un-necessarily—for no purpose—with no possible benefits. There is no risk:benefit ratio here—only risks. Every adverse reaction suffered, every side effect, every drug allergy that develops is totally unjustifiable. Every increase in bacterial resistance that occurs because of the misuse of antibiotics is unjustifiable. The bottom line is that individuals suffer from this misuse. Society suffers too, because misuse of antibiotics hastens the development of resistant strains of bacteria.

It's not just sore throats; it's every time, for whatever purpose, an antibiotic is inappropriately prescribed. So don't take antibiotics unless you understand why you need them, unless there's an identified bug that the drug is targeted to kill. There are occasions when prophylactic use of antibiotics is appropriate and necessary—for example when the gravity of the illness does not allow waiting for culture results before starting the drug. But such situations can easily be explained to you so that you can understand them. There is a logic to the use of antibiotics that you can and should understand each time you take them. If the logic isn't there, if it's not understandable, don't take the drug. In fact, whenever a treatment is proposed, whatever it is, ask enough questions to be sure that you understand it fully.

Once you begin a treatment there are other things you should know. What are the signs that it is working? How do you know if it is not? What benchmarks is your doctor following to be sure that everything is proceeding according to his plan? If your illness is marked by pain, or by swelling somewhere, or by a specific symptom you can see and monitor, how long should it be before the pain disappears, the swelling subsides, or the other symptoms abate? If you know what to expect, you can catch a treatment problem early and call it to your doctor's attention.

Many treatments fail not because the therapy is wrong but rather because it is discontinued too soon. Often, patients stop treatment when the illness stops causing the symptoms. Most of the time that will cause the problem to recur. Why? Because illness can be insidious. You're sick before you know it, before symptoms arise, and you're sick after you think you're better, after the symptoms disappear. In many cases, you may need to continue the treatment when you can't see a visible reason for it. If you understand why you need to, you're more apt to do it right.

So know what your treatment is, why it was selected from the alternatives, how it works, how to follow its progress to be sure it's doing the job, and how long it will have to be continued.

4. Questions to Ask Before Surgery Is Performed

You may find talking to your surgeon more difficult than talking to your primary care physician. After all, you didn't select him for his personality but for his technical competence. Difficult as the communication may be, however, it is absolutely essential to your health.

The first important discussion may be the hardest. It is the one where you must challenge the need for the surgery. To do this, you must ask why it is necessary and whether there are any nonsurgical alternatives. If not, ask whether other surgeons use different procedures to accomplish the same purpose. Ask the surgeon to describe exactly what he will do, so that you understand each step. And ask the surgeon to describe the risks attendant to each step.

We have already said a great deal about the need to know your surgeon's track record for the procedure, and that of the hospital in which he practices. If you haven't already checked this out before going to him, it is essential that you do so now. Directly. By asking him.

Then it gets harder. After you've challenged the need for the surgery, questioned him about his track record and that of his hospital, look him in the eye and tell him you want a second opinion. Don't worry. He really won't be offended, and he shouldn't be, because second opinions have become almost routine in the practice of surgery.

When you get a second opinion, you should be as thorough in your questions as you were with the first surgeon. You don't want a rubber stamp confirmation of what you were told. You want an independent evaluation and set of recommendations. For this reason, you should get the opinion from someone who is not an associate of the original surgeon.

One way to assure it is to begin by saying you're unconvinced about the need for surgery. Couldn't your condition get better on its own? Aren't there alternatives to surgery that should be tried first? It is always helpful if the second surgeon is not aware of the first surgeon's recommendation. He needs to know the problem of course, and that he's being asked for a second opinion. But there's no need, at the outset, for him to know what the first opinion was.

If this surgeon concurs in the need for surgery, ask him the other questions as well. See if his description of the procedures and assessment of the risks is consistent with what you were first told. Ask him what an acceptable track record would be, and what would not be acceptable. Ask him whether he knows the first surgeon's hospital, and what he thinks of it. Is his opinion based on experience or anecdote?

Finally, ask him what he thinks the consequences would be of *not* having the surgery. Sometimes when the question is put this way, it can clarify your decision. What to the surgeon would be intolerable might be no more than an inconvenience or annoyance to you—preferable to the operation and recovery. By hearing what would likely happen to you without surgery, you can make a more objective decision about what is right for you. It might be precisely correct that a condition can be cured only by surgery, but in some cases the decision to be made is not *how* to cure, but *whether* to operate. And if living with the problem uncured is acceptable to your life-style and compatible with overall good health, you may decide against surgery. For example, an operation on a bad knee might be important to someone who wants to get back to the tennis court, but irrelevant to others. One group would have the surgery; the other would not. Both would be right.

If you are persuaded that the surgery is necessary, that your surgeon is the right person for the job, and you understand what will be done to you, then it is time to move on to a different level of questions.

Before they put you to sleep, you should know what to expect when you wake up. This will help you enormously during the recovery. What will you feel like when you wake up? What is normal? What is not? Where will you be? What will be done to you? What tubes will be in you? When will your bodily functions return to working order? What are the critical benchmarks in that process? For example, when should you be making urine, and when should your G.I. system be functional? You want to know what to expect, in as much detail as you can think of to ask, so that you don't wake up and get thrown in a state of panic.

Don't wait until after the surgery to ask about the complete recuperation period. Know what to expect going in. How long will you likely be in the hospital? How long before you can go back to work? How long before you're at full strength? Knowing in advance that you face six to eight weeks of recuperation makes it a lot easier to bear. Expecting a two-week recovery when it is impossible can cause real depression or unnecessary worry. Because you've not had this operation before, you don't know what to compare it with. The goal is to know what to expect, what the benchmarks are, what the range of normal reactions includes, so that your individual experience can be put in perspective.

Sometimes things go wrong after surgery. In the immediate postoperative period, while you're in the hospital, problems are apt to be detected. Once you leave the hospital, you want to know what to be on the lookout for, so that if something happens, you can catch it quickly.

Your surgical problem may be the only medical problem you have. If so, you are fortunate. For each unrelated medical condition that you carry to the operating table potentially complicates both your surgery and your recovery. The truth is that you have to be healthy enough to undergo the trauma of surgery. Between the two extremes—too sick to withstand the operation or in perfect health except for the surgical problem—fall most patients. Be sure that your surgeon is fully aware of all other medical conditions you have, all medications you are taking, and any allergies you may have to drugs. For some medical conditions, your surgeon may want your primary care or specialty physician involved in managing the postoperative recovery on a daily basis. Whether your surgeon makes this suggestion or not, however, it's a good idea for you to ask your primary care doctor to look in on you during the postoperative period. It can't hurt, and it just might be useful. In fact, the best physicians do this as a matter of course. If they refer you to a surgeon, or if they know you are to have surgery, they will follow your case closely and visit you on their own. Why is this important? Because you want the right person for the right problem. Surgeons deal well with surgical problems. Many surgeons do less well with medical complications after surgery. You want your primary care physician or medical specialist there, following your recovery, so that he can help supervise the treatment of any medical complications. Tell that to your surgeon. Ask him to alert your physician if there's any problem, and to invite him to follow your progress in the postoperative period.

Finally, when the surgery is over and your recovery complete, make sure a full set of records is sent to your primary care physician. You might even want to get one set for yourself. For at another time, in another place, when confronted with another medical problem, showing those records may be essential to assuring that you get the best possible care.

5. Questions to Ask When a Consultant Is Called In

No matter whose idea it was to call in a consultant, you have to play an active role in selecting the individual and an equally active role in evaluating his findings and recommendations. Too often a consultant saves his detailed report for the referring doctor and gives you a light once-over. Don't let that happen. When a consultant walks into your room, don't let him walk out without answering your questions and understanding your ground rules. A consultant may not want to get between you and your doctor, may not want to be seen as in charge of your case. He doesn't want to anger the person who has called him in, and who he may hope will call him in again sometime. He may feel that how much a patient is told about the details of his case should be left up to the referring doctor. He may fear telling you more than he thinks you've already been told.

These are legitimate concerns for a consultant, but unacceptable for you. Make it clear to your primary care doctor what you expect from the consulting process. He can then tell the consultant at the outset that you are taking charge. You should then confirm this understanding with the consultant as your first order of business with him. If your doctor has not established the ground rules, do it yourself at the outset, but explain to the consultant that this approach is accepted by your primary care physician.

We have seen that consultants are called in for different purposes. What you ask the consultant depends on what the problem is.

A. *Making a diagnosis.* Ask what the physical exam, lab tests, and X rays show. Ask what the differential diagnosis is—that is, the list of possible causes of your symptoms. Which does he think is the most likely? Why? What additional tests would help him confirm his suspicion? Most important, ask him if the problem is best solved at the level of care you are presently receiving. Would additional consultants be useful? Would a university setting make more sense? At what point would the next level of care be appropriate? You want to get a feel for how much trouble you're in. Some problems are very difficult to diagnose but the consequences of either never succeeding, or of any of the possibilities being confirmed, are relatively minor. That is, no matter what the cause is, it won't kill you, disable you, or significantly affect your functioning. Other problems are both difficult to diagnose and, depending on which of several alternatives is the cause, may have profound, life-threatening consequences. Symptoms can be initially misleading; they may be severe even though the problem is, in fact, relatively minor. You're looking for an assessment from the consultant as to where on the spectrum you fall. Then you can decide if you're being treated at the appropriate level of care. In other words, the consultant should be used not only to help solve the problem, but also to help decide where the best place would be to solve the problem. The consultant may be reluctant to recommend transferring you to another facility because that would mean transferring responsibility for your case away from your primary care doctor. So you must raise the issue yourself. And push him on it. He may laugh and assure you that where you are is more than adequate to handle your problem; but if he's really concerned about you, and if you give him this opportunity to comment, he will find it easier to recommend a transfer up the line. In some cases, the need for a university setting is obvious; at other times, it might be preferable, but is probably not essential. It is those cases—where you *could* be treated where you are but it is clearly *better* to be treated elsewhere—that you will uncover by pushing your consultant. If it's your illness, or your loved one's, "clearly better" will prevail every time.

B. *Advising a treatment.* When deciding on a treatment for an already diagnosed problem, your questions will be slightly different. You want to know what the alternatives are, how they work to solve your problem, and what risks are entailed in each case. It's useful to find out if a scientific consensus exists on the best treatment for the problem at hand, or whether several different approaches are in vogue, perhaps different ones in different parts of the country. Ask if there is any active, promising research in this area, and what, if any, experimental treatments are being evaluated. By asking these questions, you will occasionally find a doctor who says, "The conventional way of treating this is 'A' but I've had much better success with 'B.' " If you hear that, beware. He might be right, but the burden of proof should be on him to demonstrate to you and your primary care doctor why his way is better than almost everyone else's.

There are doctors who use outmoded, even discredited therapies; some are slow to change even after the world of medicine has passed them by. But others are at the frontiers of medicine, developing the accepted treatments of tomorrow. You need to know which kind of doctor your consultant is.

You must also probe the question of which level of care your problem needs. You need to know if you are at the right place to have the recommended treatment administered most effectively.

When a treatment has been proposed and accepted, ask the consultant how it should be carried out and monitored. How will you know if it is succeeding or failing? What should you watch out for? What are the early warning signs of possible trouble?

C. *Evaluating a treatment failure.* Nothing is more frustrating than thinking a problem is solved, and finding that it persists. The diagnosis is made. The treatment is carried out. You don't get any better. Enter the consultant. In such cases you want to be sure that the diagnosis itself is correct. Ask the consultant if he concurs, and whether another factor, in addition to what has been diagnosed, is at work in your case.

If the diagnosis is clear but the treatment is not working, you want your consultant to set it straight. You also want him to assess whether the problem should have happened at all. In other words, do you need to replace your original physician? Because he has been called in by that physician, the consultant will be very reluctant to discuss him. But you can approach it indirectly, by probing how the error, if there was one, was made.

Many times treatments fail not because of physician error but because of the complexities of the particular case, or the failure of the patient to adhere properly to the regimen. Ask the consultant what changes are necessary, and why. What other alternatives exist? Why is this approach likely to succeed when the other has failed? You may find, in response, that several different approaches need to be tried in order to find the one that works. In that case, review very carefully the risks of the alternatives so that you can, all things being equal, try the least risky one first. If your doctor proposes a different order, be sure there are solid reasons for believing that the riskier approach also has the greatest chance of success. Ask him to explain the basis for that conclusion to be sure it is more than anecdotal experience.

Again, it is very important to determine whether, in view of the treatment failure, you're at the best place in the health care system to find a solution.

Whatever the purpose of the consultation, when it is over you should compare notes with your primary doctor. Be sure that his understanding of what was found and recommended is the same as yours. It's a good idea, whenever possible, to end the consultation with a group meeting with you, your doctor, and your consultant. That way everyone can hear the same thing at the same time. In such settings, it is very useful to expose any difference that may exist between the two physicians. Hearing them discuss it together may help you to evaluate what to do about the disagreement. The fact is, though, the overwhelming majority of the time, this kind of disagreement should lead you to obtain yet another opinion.

6. Questions to Ask When You Are Seriously Ill and Told, "There's Nothing More to Be Done"

"How much time have I got left?" A difficult question to ask. An impossible one to answer. For in most cases, there is no way to predict.

Every doctor has a point at which he will give up, when he will say there's nothing more he can do. This is the hardest of all times to think about taking charge, but it is the time when taking charge can have the greatest impact on your life. It can literally save it. For when a doctor says there is nothing more he can do, it's not necessarily true that nothing more can be done by anyone.

The fact is that different doctors give up at different times and for different reasons. When a doctor says that there's nothing more to be done, it really means there's nothing more to be done *by him,* or the colleagues and consultants he knows. Whether there's something that someone else can do must be explored.

Never accept someone else's judgment that you've reached the end of the line, that there are no more options left. You must come to that judgment by yourself, after you have fought as hard as you can to find out if there's someone, somewhere, who just might be able to help.

I have several close friends who are alive today because they refused to give up when their doctors did. When their doctors walked away, they began to fight.

If your doctor says there's no more to be done, as difficult as it may be, ask him to explain why. Make sure you understand the problem. Ask him if he's talked to his colleagues or consulted with the known experts in the disease. Ask whether there is active research going on in this area, or whether any experimental treatment programs exist. Tell him you understand he may be right, but you want to pursue it further, and ask where he thinks you should go for another evaluation. Make it clear to him that you're not quite ready to give up.

What can be gained from this conversation? Surely if he knew of anyone else to consult or anything else to try, he would have done it already, right? Wrong. He might have; he might in fact be correct in his assessment of your situation. But he might not have. He might have made a value judgment about not putting you through more tests, more treatments, more operations, because the slim chance of success was outweighed by the difficulties and risks of the treatment. He might have made the value judgment that your quality of remaining life should not be sacrificed for so little chance of success. But it's not his value judgment to make. It's yours. What he thinks is right for you, or reasonable to do, cannot substitute for what you think. Confronted with death, the quality of your remaining life may be far less important to you than taking any chance, any risk, no matter how unpleasant, in order to prolong your life.

The purpose of the conversation is for you to fully understand the basis of his giving up, to be sure that "nothing more to be done" doesn't mean "nothing more that in my judgment would be reasonable for you to do." Sometimes, when it's clear to him that you intend to press on, he will reenlist in the effort. In other situations, he will help find the best place to go to give it one last-ditch try.

Most of the time, when your doctor gives up it is with good reason. Most of the time, in fact, he will be right—there will be nothing else to do. But *most of the time* is not necessarily *your time,* so ask the questions, get another evaluation, and hope for the best.

HOW TO REACH
THE FRONTIERS OF MEDICINE

When a doctor has done everything he knows for you, there may still be more that can be done: things that he doesn't yet know about because they are being developed at the frontiers of medicine. It may be years before your doctor learns of treatments being given today by clinical researchers in university hospitals. Your job, your challenge, is to find that frontier for your problem and, if it exists, find where it is and how you get to it.

The stakes are very high. If you have a chronic, disabling disease or one that threatens your life, help may be found only in a handful of institutions in the country. It may seem like trying to find a needle in a haystack. How do you do it?

The process is a lot like finding the right medical specialist. Start by asking your doctor to put you in touch with a university-based specialist in the disease. You may, in fact, already have used him as a consultant. He may be someone with great experience and skill who has mastered all the known and accepted approaches to your problem. You're talking to him now for a different purpose, however, because you want to find out where, if anywhere, the untested but promising treatments of tomorrow are being developed. You want to know who the top researchers in the country are and whether anyone, anywhere, is trying something different. He may know; he may not. He may assure you he's aware of the latest developments in the field and has already considered them. He may in fact be right. But you can't stop there. You must confirm that judgment for yourself. Why? Because a lot of work goes on at the frontier before the results are published, before scientific papers are presented at professional meetings—in other words, before even top-flight university specialists become aware of it.

Almost all such research at the frontier is funded by an organization. You must locate these funding sources and find out whether relevant experimental work is under way, and if so, where. By far, the largest such funding source is the federal government. And the place to start is the National Institutes of Health in Bethesda, Maryland.

The awarding of public money for research grants is public information. You are entitled to it. So phone the appropriate Institute at NIH and ask whether any research relevant to your problem is being supported, and if it is, who is carrying it out. Sometimes by listening to your problem, an NIH staff member can direct you to the most promising possibilities; at other times, you will have to check everyone on the list. When you have this information, ask your doctor to make the calls. If your problem is cancer, your doctor should start with the *PDQ* system. Even with cancer, however, a follow-up phone call to the Cancer Institute is worthwhile if no new leads emerge from *PDQ*.

NIH operates its own clinical center at the Bethesda, Maryland campus, where high quality, experimental treatment research goes on every day. Find out if one of the research studies is relevant to your problem. If it is, find out the procedure for getting accepted into this experimental treatment program. This is not always a simple matter because the main purpose of the research projects is clinical investigation rather than treating patients. In some studies, in fact, half the patients will not get the experimental drug at all, only a placebo. You may not fit the experimental criteria, and the number of people seeking entry may be far greater than the size of the program. Moreover, NIH decisions are often influenced by politics. Congressmen have clout with NIH because they vote on its funds, and NIH tries, whenever possible, to accommodate them. It's a bias in the system that you can't successfully fight. So fight fire with fire and enlist your own congressmen and senators in the effort to get you admitted.

The government isn't the only source of funding for research. You should turn to private organizations, like the American Cancer Society and the Muscular Dystrophy Association of America, for help. These groups usually know what is going on, and where, even if it is funded by another group.

The pharmaceutical industry is a major source of funding for clinical research around the world. Unlike government studies, however, research by private companies is often a closely guarded secret. Companies don't want competitors to know what they're working on, particularly early in the research process. While it may be impossible to find out what's going on in their basic research laboratories, you need to know what the companies are doing in testing specific drugs and treatments. Before a new drug can be approved by the FDA, it has to undergo extensive clinical trials, many of which are carried out by university specialists who are expert in the field. In these trials, patients are given the new drug or treatment for the first time to see if it is safe and then if it works. If the experimental drug is designed for your particular problem, you may want to try to get into those trials.

How do you find out what drug or treatment is being tested, and where? If there is a clinical trial under way, it is part of the FDA's regulatory process. Have your doctor call the FDA, describe the problem, and ask if clinical trials are underway that might be of help. At certain stages of development, experimental drugs can be made available to individual doctors for use with particular patients. You may be that patient. Your doctor will have to fill out detailed forms for the FDA, but it's a way of getting you a treatment that might not be generally known or available for months or even years.

The other approach is to go directly to the pharmaceutical companies. Because profits depend on how many times doctors prescribe their products, the companies are very receptive to doctors' requests. If you learn which company is conducting the relevant clinical trials, have your doctor call to try to get you into the trial. Or, with the company's help, he can initiate the paperwork required by the FDA to allow him to obtain the drug for you.

If you don't know which company is conducting the trials, and the FDA is not very helpful, have your doctor call the Pharmaceutical Manufacturers Association in Washington, D.C. If he describes the problem and the urgency of your situation, the staff may be able to tell him which of their member companies is working on relevant new drugs.

There is no guarantee that successfully reaching the frontiers of medicine will solve your problem. The sad truth is that more often than not, it won't. After all, the frontier is a unique place, a place of trial and error, of high promise and grave disappointment. Theories are tested. Some are confirmed; others refuted. Some new treatments succeed; others fail. The risks to you are great because much less is known about what to expect. And yet all progress, all advances in medicine, originate at the frontier. And then they slowly filter down to every level of the health care system.

Is it worth the effort to reach the frontier? There are people who are alive today only because they made that effort, after their original doctors had given up. Others reached it and had their lives end in pain and suffering. Whether it is worth it to you depends on how hard you want to fight, how much you want a victory. Doctors are not the only ones who give up at different times. Patients do too. Your decision depends on many things: how much pain you're in, how impaired your functioning is, what the quality of life has been for you, how much more you are prepared to endure. No one can answer those questions for you. There is no right or wrong. But at the very least, you should know what options exist. And one of them is to try to reach the frontier.

AIDS

Plague. The very sound of the word is frightening. It conjures up visions of a microscopic killer on the loose destroying millions of defenseless men, women, and children.

We live in an uneasy balance with the microbes that are all around us. That has always been true, and AIDS teaches us once again that it always will be true.

Microbes move where man moves. When civilizations were isolated from one another, each was protected from some of the unique hazards that afflicted the others. When explorers set sail, they carried not only high hopes but also dangerous microbes. When Captain Cook sailed the Pacific and came ashore on the western side of Kauai, he brought not only the flag, blankets, and gifts to the natives; he also brought syphilis, and in short order the majority of the population of native Hawaiians was dead. And that story of the inadvertent transmission of deadly disease from place to place was replicated all over the world.

It is easy to forget how delicate the balance really is. Before the antibiotic era dawned in the 1940s, and before vaccines were perfected, doctors could diagnose many life-threatening diseases that they couldn't treat. Death sentences were pronounced every day, with words like tuberculosis, diphtheria, pneumonia, rheumatic fever, influenza, yellow fever, typhoid fever, tetanus. In those days, what you had was clear. What it could do to you was clear. What you could do about it was . . . nothing.

Today we have antibiotics. We have vaccines. We even have a few antiviral agents. But we still live with the uneasy balance. There are still microbial diseases we can recognize but not cure. And there always will be.

Why? Because both sides of the balance are changing all the time. The microbes themselves change. The flu virus comes out with new models all the time, and just for good measure it recycles the old ones at periodic intervals. Other viruses mutate and become more, or less, of a threat. New diseases arise as a result. Bacteria change. They respond to the weapons we direct at them and become resistant. We have to change these weapons continually to keep up. Bacteria have to expand their resistance to survive. It is an uneasy balance, with everything always changing.

As we live longer, we face new and different problems. The diseases of middle age—heart attack, high blood pressure, many forms of cancer—could not show themselves in populations that lived only into their thirties. And we still don't know what causes all our diseases, or how to treat them. We are just beginning to learn that microbes may be attacking us in ways we never suspected, causing problems we never attributed to them. Certain forms of cancer, for example, are now being linked to viruses.

Every advance we make is countered by a response, or by the emergence of a new problem. And yet our basic direction is forward. We live with the balance, but we live longer, healthier lives. New problems arise. Some of them are frightening. They exact a dreadful toll of suffering and death, but eventually we solve them, only to face the next challenge. The delicate balance remains.

AIDS is the most pressing current challenge. It is frightening. It exacts a dreadful toll of suffering and death. Yet, at some point, AIDS will be successfully overcome. That we will achieve success is certain. *When* is not. We live today in the uncertain interval between the promise and the cure.

How long will it last? No one knows. By historical standards, not very long at all. But for you and me, and all those with loved ones at risk, the interval will seem endless. During this time, we will witness the deaths of tens of thousands of men, women, and children. We will see communities divide over how to treat the victims in their midst. We will see examples of extraordinary compassion and understanding side by side with examples of unconscionable callousness and persecution. We will see the best in us and the worst.

How can one take charge when the disease is AIDS? We will have to understand what is known and what is not; what is fact and what is myth; what places one at risk and what lessens or eliminates risk; what treatments exist, what they can do, and what their limitations are.

Let's be clear about one thing: What we know is always chang-ing, ever expanding. You will know far more when you read this page than you could have when the page was written. Whatever is known is quickly outdated. But until a cure or preventive vaccine is developed, no matter how much more is known, some things will not change. AIDS will remain a death sentence for all infected with it. As many as 270,000 cases may be reported in this country by 1991, with 179,000 deaths by that year.[1]

With statistics like these, and no current remedy available to alter them, what is known will be of little comfort to the victim, and it will have to compete with what is myth. The most pernicious example is the myth of a miracle cure being suppressed by the medical establishment, lurking somewhere in the medical underground, perhaps just beyond the borders in Mexico. When the medical profession says it can do nothing, desperate people, fighting for their lives, will try anything. At any cost. And often they end up losing their lives as well as their money. For there is an industry of vultures who prey upon the terminally ill, promising them miracles but delivering dashed hopes and exorbitant bills. So it is important to know the facts—and avoid the frauds.

With statistics like these, there is also a tendency to trumpet each legitimate scientific advance, to overstate it, to raise hopes prematurely. The wish becomes father to the thought. A new drug is developed. Rumors about it sweep the network of victims and their families. A clamor for its instant approval begins in the press. The Food and Drug Administration, under great pressure, approves the substance without requiring the usual data available for review. In so doing, it warns that the drug has real risks, is not for everyone, that for pre-AIDS (ARC) syndrome, or nonadvanced AIDS, the risks far outweigh the benefits. But the warnings tend to get lost in the hoopla as the press reports the first AIDS drug on the market. Every victim wants it. Doctors are pressured to prescribe it, even when they shouldn't. Can they withstand the pressure? What do you think?

Is this an imaginary case? No, it is a summary of the story of AZT, the first drug actually approved by the FDA for use in AIDS. Does it cure AIDS? No, not even close. It does prolong short-term survival for some seriously ill AIDS patients, but it is too toxic to be safely used by all AIDS patients. Better than nothing? For some patients, surely. But not for every stage of the disease. In fact, it can be a lot worse than nothing.

The bottom line: If you have AIDS, you have to know what's so and what isn't so. You have to be able to separate myth from reality, to use what can help *in the stage in which it can help*. There will be new developments all the time. Know what they are, and what they are not; what they can really do, and what they can't. These developments can't be described here very effectively because they will be so quickly outdated. That is, in fact, the good news. There's a lot going on. The goal is to play for time, to slow things down, to hope for a breakthrough. And to come to terms with yourself.

What if you don't have AIDS? What is the purpose of taking charge? To avoid it. And you can. Absolutely. Because it is a matter of personal choice—whether to risk getting the disease at all, or how much risk to take.

We know what causes AIDS. We know how to test for it in your body. We know how AIDS is transmitted. Most important, we know how to prevent the spread of AIDS to you. Whether you choose to act on what we know is up to you. Because we can't yet cure the disease or biologically prevent it through vaccines, and because if you get it, you will almost certainly die from it, your decision about risk is literally a life-and-death proposition.

As of this writing, here is what we know: The AIDS virus can be recovered from an infected person's blood, semen, vaginal fluid, tears, and saliva. It has been shown to be transmitted, however, only through blood, semen, and vaginal secretions.

The risk derives from the method of transmission. If you have no intimate contact with infected blood, semen, or vaginal secretion, you will have no chance of getting AIDS. It's that simple. And that difficult.

Before we knew what AIDS was or how to test for it, the virus infiltrated the nation's blood supply. Some patients needing transfusions got something with the blood that they didn't need at all—infection with AIDS. Today we can screen donated blood for the virus. We do, routinely, and our blood supply is much safer. Not perfectly safe, because the screening process does not detect the virus in the days immediately following initial infection. To minimize risk, the blood you receive should be your own, donated prior to surgery, or from donors you know well and feel confident do not have AIDS.

The blood of intravenous drug users who share needles is far from safe. The infection precedes the knowledge of the infection. When the needles are shared, the disease is passed from addict to addict through contaminated blood. So AIDS is a disease of addicts, of intravenous drug users.

AIDS is also a venereal disease. Like all venereal diseases, it is a potential risk for everyone. And like all venereal diseases, it is a particular risk for young adults who are already experiencing an explosion of sexually transmitted diseases. AIDS can be spread from man to man, man to woman, or woman to man. And in spite of all the publicity, all the warnings, in spite of the knowledge that infection means death, AIDS continues to spread as a result of individual choice and individual decisions to take chances, as venereal diseases have spread since the beginning of time.

No one can tell you how to live your life; we can only show you your risks of ending it.

Modern technology can certify you as AIDS-free. A monogamous sexual relationship with another AIDS-free individual will eliminate your risk entirely. Beyond that, it's a matter of degree of risk. Do you want to know about your partner—for sure? It's possible to find out. Can't wait or don't want to ask? The risk increases. Multiple sex partners? Multiple risk. How to reduce the risk? Physical barriers to prevent contact with possibly infected fluids: condoms with spermicides. Are they guaranteed to work? No. Are condoms better than nothing? Yes, a whole lot better. Does this advice apply to gay men and women as well as heterosexuals? Of course it does. The disease is epidemic in these communities because the transmission is biologically easier with anal sex, because the populations are more concentrated in certain areas, and because the disease took hold and spread widely before it was recognized or understood. But AIDS is not a "gay person's disease." It's a danger to everyone, and each of us can choose to prevent it.

Individual choice. The difference between life and death. Sounds melodramatic, but it isn't. It's a fact. There's one other individual choice to be aware of as well, an equally important one. If you are a female and have AIDS, there is a very real risk, if you become pregnant, of giving birth to a baby infected with AIDS. It has happened, too many times. Your baby has no choice. If you're infected, you do. Don't get pregnant.

What makes the AIDS story so frightening right now is the virtual certainty of death for all infected with it. And the fact that the virus took such a firm foothold all around us before we knew it was there. What is remarkable, however, is not that a disease of such virulence sneaked up on us, but rather that we detected it so quickly. More definitive medical treatment and biological prevention are certain to follow. In the interim, taking charge can have real benefit in helping AIDS patients plan for time. AZT can help some extend and improve the quality of their lives now. Newer drugs will become available that will help even more—maybe even buy enough time to allow survival until a cure is found.

We cannot escape the uneasy balance with the microbes all around us. There will be other epidemics, some more virulent, some less. It has happened since the beginning of time. The AIDS virus itself may change, in significant or trivial ways. The challenge is to respond quickly each time. We can't escape the temporary imbalance new dangers present. We can only restore the uneasy balance as rapidly as possible to minimize the damage.

NOTES

HOSPITALS: HYSTERECTOMY AND CESAREAN SECTION

1. John Wennberg and Alan Gittelsohn, "Variations in Medical Care Among Small Areas," *Scientific American* 246:120–34, April 1982.

2. John E. Wennberg, John P. Bunker, and Benjamin Barnes, "The Need for Assessing the Outcome of Common Medical Practices," *Annual Review of Public Health* 1:277–95, 1980.

3. Alexander M. Walker and Hershel Jick, "Temporal and Regional Variation in Hysterectomy Rates in the United States, 1970–1975," *American Journal of Epidemiology* 110:41–6, July 1979.

4. Thomas D. Koepsell, Noel S. Weiss, Donovan J. Thompson, et al., "Prevalence of Prior Hysterectomy in the Seattle-Tacoma Area," *American Journal of Public Health* 70:40–7, January 1980.

5. Nancy C. Lee, Richard C. Dicker, George L. Rubin, et al., "Confirmation of the Preoperative Diagnoses for Hysterectomy," *American Journal of Obstetrics and Gynecology* 150:283–7, October 1984.

6. J. M. Grant and I. Y. Hussein, "An Audit of Abdominal Hysterectomy Over a Decade in a District Hospital," *British Journal of Obstetrics and Gynecology* 91: 73–7, January 1984.

7. National Center for Health Statistics, "Midwife and Out-of-Hospital Deliveries," National Vital Statistics System Series 21, No. 40, February 1984.

8. Paul J. Placek, Selma Taffel, and Mary Moien, "Cesarean Section Delivery Rates: United States, 1981," *American Journal of Public Health* 73:861–2, August 1983.

9. Marion H. Hall, "When a Woman Asks for a Caesarean Section," *British Medical Journal* 294:201–2, January 1987.

10. George L. Rubin, Herbert B. Peterson, Roger W. Rochat, et al., "Maternal Death After Cesarean Section in Georgia," *American Journal of Obstetrics and Gynecology* 139:681–5, March 1981.

11. Thorkild F. Nielsen and Klas-Henry Hökegård, "Postoperative Cesarean Section Morbidity: A Prospective Study," *American Journal of Obstetrics and Gynecology* 146:911–6, August 1983.

12. O. Hunter Jones, "Cesarean Section in Present-Day Obstetrics," *American Journal of Obstetrics and Gynecology* 126:521–30, November 1976.

13. Sidney F. Bottoms, Mortimer G. Rosen, and Robert J. Sokol, "The Increase in the Cesarean Birth Rate," *New England Journal of Medicine* 302:559–63, March 1980.

14. Joseph V. Collea, Connie Chein, and Edward J. Quilligan, "The Randomized Management of Term Frank Breech Presentation: A Study of 208 Cases," *American Journal of Obstetrics and Gynecology* 137:235–44, May 1980.

CANCER

1. Division of Cancer Prevention and Control, National Cancer Institute, *1985 Annual Cancer Statistics Review*, NIH Publ. No. 86-2789 (Bethesda, Md., December 1985).

2. A fascinating account of the history of the Halsted procedure can be found in Jay Katz's book *The Silent World of Doctor and Patient* (New York: Free Press, 1984).

3. "Breast Cancer," from April 22, 1986, inquiry to the *Physician Data Query (PDQ)*, a computer database for physicians, National Cancer Institute, International Cancer Information Center, Bethesda, Maryland.

4. Barbara J. Culliton, "Information as a 'Cure' for Cancer," *Science* 227:732, February 1985.

5. "Cancer Deaths, Dosages Tied," *Washington Post*, March 25, 1986, p. A5.

6. Patricia K. Duffner, Michael E. Cohen, and John T. Flannery, "Referral Patterns of Childhood Brain Tumors in the State of Connecticut," *Cancer* 50:1636–40, October 1982.

7. Maurice Griffel, "Wilms' Tumor in New York State: Epidemiology and Survivorship," *Cancer* 40:3140–5, December 1977.

8. Gerald E. Hanks, James J. Diamond, and Simon Kramer, "The Need for Complex Technology in Radiation Oncology: Correlations of Facility Characteristics and Structure with Outcome," *Cancer* 55:2198–201, May 1985.

9. Jeanne J. Kinzie, Gerald E. Hanks, Charles J. Maclean, et al., "Patterns of Care Study: Hodgkin's Disease Relapse Rates and Adequacy of Portals," *Cancer* 52:2223–6, December 1983.

10. Gerald E. Hanks, David F. Herring, and Simon Kramer, "Patterns of Care Outcome Studies: Results of the National Practice in Cancer of the Cervix," *Cancer* 51:959–67, March 1983.

HEART DISEASE

1. Charles B. Christian, Jr., John W. Mack, and Lewis Wetstein, "Current Status of Coronary Artery Bypass Grafting for Coronary Artery Atherosclerosis," *Surgical Clinics of North America* 65:509–26, June 1985.

2. Thomas B. Graboys, Adrienne Headley, Bernard Lown, et al., "Results of a Second-Opinion Program for Coronary Artery Bypass Graft Surgery," *Journal of the American Medical Association* 258:1611–4, September 1987.

3. Harold S. Luft and Sandra S. Hunt, "Evaluating Individual Hospital Quality Through Outcome Statistics," *Journal of the American Medical Association* 255: 2780–4, May 1986.

4. Lisa M. Krieger, "Diagnostic Tool May Be Fatal," *San Francisco Examiner*, October 11, 1987, p. A4.

5. Louis R. Caplan, "Carotid-Artery Disease" (editorial), *New England Journal of Medicine* 315:886–8, October 1986.

6. Brian R. Chambers and John W. Norris, "Outcome in Patients with Asymptomatic Neck Bruits," *New England Journal of Medicine* 315:860–5, October 1986.

7. Paul Leren and Anders Helgeland, "Coronary Heart Disease and Treatment of Hypertension: Some Oslo Study Data," *American Journal of Medicine Supplement* 80(2A):3–6, February 1986.

8. Myron H. Weinberger, "Antihypertensive Therapy and Lipids: Paradoxical Influences on Cardiovascular Disease Risk," *American Journal of Medicine Supplement* 80(2A):64–70, February 1986.

9. Mark V. Pauly, "The Changing Health Care Environment," *American Journal of Medicine Supplement* 81(6C):3–8, December 1986.

10. William B. Stason, "Opportunities for Improving the Cost-Effectiveness of Antihypertensive Treatment," *American Journal of Medicine Supplement* 81(6C):45–9, December 1986.

DRUGS

1. Steven H. Erickson, James J. Bergman, Ronald Schneeweiss, et al., "The Use of Drugs for Unlabeled Indications," *Journal of the American Medical Association* 243:1543–6, April 1980.

2. Brian L. Strom, Kenneth L. Melmon, Olli S. Miettinen, "Post-Marketing Studies of Drug Efficacy: Why?" *American Journal of Medicine* 78:475–80, March 1985.

3. Duane M. Kirking, J. William Thomas, Frank J. Ascione, et al., "Detecting and Preventing Adverse Drug Interactions: The Potential Contribution of Computers in Pharmacies," *Social Science & Medicine* 22:1–8, 1986.

4. D. Price, J. Cooke, S. Singleton, et al., "Doctors' Unawareness of the Drugs Their Patients Are Taking: A Major Cause of Overprescribing?" *British Medical Journal* 292:99–100, January 1986.

5. Phil R. Manning, Peter V. Lee, William A. Clintworth, et al., "Changing Prescribing Practices Through Individual Continuing Education," *Journal of the American Medical Association* 256:230–2, July 1986.

LABORATORY TESTS: HOW MUCH IS ENOUGH?

1. Lois P. Myers and Steven A. Schroeder, "Physician Use of Services for the Hospitalized Patient: A Review, with Implications for Cost Containment," *Milbank Memorial Fund Quarterly* 59:481–507, Summer 1981.

2. Steven A. Schroeder, Kathryn Kenders, James K. Cooper, et al., "Use of Laboratory Tests and Pharmaceuticals: Variation Among Physicians and Effect of Cost Audit on Subsequent Use," *Journal of the American Medical Association* 255:-969–73, August 1973.

3. Arnold M. Epstein, Robert M. Hartley, John R. Charlton, et al., "A Comparison of Ambulatory Test Ordering for Hypertensive Patients in the United States and England," *Journal of the American Medical Association* 252:1723–6, October 1984.

4. Robert M. Hartley, Arnold M. Epstein, Conrad M. Harris, et al., "Differences in Ambulatory Test Ordering in England and America: Role of Doctors' Beliefs and Attitudes," *American Journal of Medicine* 82:513–7, March 1987.

5. D. Joe Boone, Hugh J. Hansen, Thomas L. Hearn, et al., "Laboratory Evaluation and Assistance Efforts: Mailed, On-Site and Blind Proficiency Testing Surveys Conducted by the Centers for Disease Control," *American Journal of Public Health* 72:1364–8, December 1982.

6. Charles W. Griffin III, Mary A. Mehaffey, Ellen C. Cook, et al., "Relationship Between Performance in Three of the Centers for Disease Control Microbiology Proficiency Testing Programs and the Number of Actual Patient Specimens Tested by Participating Laboratories," *Journal of Clinical Microbiology* 23:246–50, February 1986.

7. Robert Crawley, Richard Belsey, Darrell Brock, et al., "Regulation of Physicians' Office Laboratories: The Idaho Experience," *Journal of the American Medical Association* 255:374–82, January 1986.

THE CASE FOR TAKING CHARGE

1. From *Physician Characteristics and Distribution in the U.S.*, 1986 ed., OP-180/5 (American Medical Association, P.O. Box 10946, Chicago, IL 60610).

2. 1984 data obtained from the Federation of State Medical Boards of the U.S., Inc. (2630 W. Freeway, Suite 138, Fort Worth, TX 76102).

OBSTACLES TO TAKING CHARGE

1. Jay Katz, *The Silent World of Doctor and Patient* (New York: Free Press, 1984), p. xiii.

2. Ibid., p. 2.

NOTES

HOW TO TAKE CHARGE

1. Rhonda L. Rundle, "Hospitals Cite Mortality Statistics in Ads to Attract Heart Patients," *Wall Street Journal*, July 28, 1987, p. 25.

AIDS

1. "Confronting AIDS: Directions for Public Health, Health Care and Research," Institute of Medicine, 1986.

APPENDIX 1: TELEPHONE NUMBERS FOR THE NATIONAL INSTITUTES OF HEALTH

	Inst.	Phone	Bldg.
Clinical Center	CC	496-2563	10-1C255
Division of Computer Resource Technology	DCRT	496-6203	12A-3027
Division of Research Grants	DRG	496-7441	WW-448
Division of Research Resources	DRR	496-5545	31-5B10
Division of Research Services	DRS	496-5795	12A-4007
Fogarty International Center	FIC	496-2075	16-210
National Cancer Institute	NCI	496-6631	31-10A29
		496-5583	31-10A18
National Eye Institute	NEI	496-5248	31-6A32
National Heart, Lung, Blood Institute	NHLBI	496-4236	31-4A21
National Institute of Aging	NIA	496-1752	31-5C35
Allergies & Infectious Disease	NIAID	496-5717	31-7A32
Arthritis	NIAMS	496-8188	31-B2B15E
Child Health	NICHD	496-5133	31-2A34
Diabetes, Digestion & Kidney	NIDDK	496-3583	31-9A04
Dental Research	NIDR	496-4261	31-2C35
Environmental Health	NIEHS		P.O. Box
	(919) 541-3345		12233,
	8-629-3345		Research Triangle, NC 27709
General Medicine	NIGMS	496-7301	31-4A52
Mental Health	NIMH	443-4536	Parklawn
		443-4513	15-102
		496-1678	Jules Bldg.
Neurological Communicable Diseases & Stroke	NINCDS	496-5924	31-8A06
		496-5751	31-8A16
Library of Medicine	NLM	496-6308	38-2S-10

OFFICE OF THE DIRECTOR (OD) STAFF

496-2433	1 -124	Dr. James B. Wyngaarden	Director
496-2121	1 -132	Dr. William F. Raub	Deputy Director
496-1921	1 -122	Dr. Joseph E. Rall	Deputy Director for Intramural Research
496-1096	1 -107	Dr. Katherine L. Bick	Deputy Director for Extraramural Research
496-5356	1 -111	Dr. George J. Galasso	Associate Director for Extramural Affairs
496-4466	1 -136	John D. Mahoney	Associate Director for Administration
496-2215	1 -118	Dr. Edwin D. Becker	Associate Director for Research Services
496-3561	1 -103	Dr. Philip S. Chen	Associate Director for Intramural Affairs
496-4461	1 -309	Storm Whaley	Associate Director for Communications

Information Officer	Director	Phone	Bldg.
Irene Haske	Dr. John L. Decker	496-4114	10-2C146
Patricia Miller	Dr. Arnold Pratt	496-5703	12A-3033
Dr. Sam Joseloff	Dr. Jerome G. Green	496-7211	WB-450
James Augustine	Dr. Betty Pickett	496-9567	31-5B03
James Doherty	Dr. Robert Whitney, Jr.	496-5793	12A-4007
Jim Bryant	Dr. Craig Wallace	496-1415	38A-605
Eleanor Nealon	Dr. Vincent DeVita, Jr.	496-5615	31-11A52
Public Inquiries			
Mary Lynn Hendrix	Dr. Carl Kupfer	496-2234	31-6A03
Terry Bellicha	Dr. Claude Lenfant	496-5166	31-5A52
Jane Shure	Dr. T. Franklin Williams	496-9265	31-2C02
Pat Randall	Dr. Anthony S. Fauci	496-2263	31-7A03
Connie Raab	Dr. Lawrence E. Shulman	496-4353	31-9A35
Michaela Richardson	Dr. Duane Alexander	496-3454	31-2A03
Betsy Singer	Dr. Phillip Gorden	496-5877	31-9A52
Brent Jaquet	Dr. Harald Loe	496-3571	31-2C39
Hugh Lee	Dr. David Rall	(8-629-3201)	
		(919) 541-3201	
Ann Dieffenbach	Dr. Ruth Kirschstein	496-5231	31-4A52
Ed Long	Dr. Shervert Frazier	443-3673	Parklawn
Public Inquiries			17-99
International			
Sylvia Shaffer	Dr. Murray Goldstein	496-3167	31-8A52
Public Inquiries			
Robert Mehnert	Dr. Donald Lindberg	496-6221	38A-7N707

OFFICE OF THE DIRECTOR (OD) STAFF *(Continued)*

496-3553	1 -132	Dr. Vida Beaven	Assistant Director for Program Coordination
496-4114	10-2C146	Dr. John L. Decker	Associate Director for Clinical Care
496-3152	1 -137	Dr. Jay Moskowitz	Associate Director for Program Planning & Evaluation
496-1508	1 -216	Dr. William Friedewald	Associate Director for Disease Prevention
496-1143	1 -210	Dr. Itzhak Jacoby	Acting Director, Office of Medical Application of Research
496-4920	1 -101	Dr. John C. Eberhart	Senior Advisor to Deputy Director for Intramural Research
496-1318	1 -10	Dr. Karen P. O'Steen	Executive Secretariat Director
496-4713	1 -313	Thomas Flavin	Special Projects Officer
496-5163	1 -119	OD FILES	

APPENDIX 2:
PDQ SYSTEM

This is a sample of a *PDQ* System printout. Though this particular selection refers to breast cancer, similar information is available to physicians for a wide variety of illnesses. Show this section to your physician, whatever your illness, as an example of how the system can be utilized.

start

NXM.USER.NCI11.DATA   On PRIV85 as SNCI11 SEQ OLD

THE NATIONAL LIBRARY OF MEDICINE WELCOMES YOU TO
THE NATIONAL CANCER INSTITUTE'S PDQ SYSTEM

Date: 01/27/88   Time: 1:54 pm EST

PDQ ACCESS is now available for IBM, Compaq and IBM-compatible personal computers. See PDQ NEWS for details.

Note: See news item 5 for important changes in Protocol retrieval.

*Press CR to continue.

>

PDQ MENU

The following information is available in PDQ.

1 Description	5 Physicians
2 Instructions	6 Organizations
3 News	7 Protocols (See news item 5)
4 Cancer Information	8 PDQ Editorial Board

9 Exit PDQ

At any PDQ prompt (>), you may type HELP to obtain assistance with your PDQ search.

*Enter desired number and press CR ("Return" or "Enter" key).

> 4

Diagnosis selection

1 By body system/site
2 By histologic tissue/type
3 By childhood cancer

*Enter desired number OR type in a diagnosis and press CR.

> 1

DIAGNOSIS SELECTION BY BODY SYSTEM/SITE

1 Acquired immune deficiency syndrome (AIDS)
2 Breast
3 Digestive/gastrointestinal
4 Endocrine
5 Eye
6 Female reproductive
7 Head and neck
8 Hematological
9 Kidney/urinary
10 Male reproductive
11 Musculoskeletal

12 Neurological

13 Skin

14 Thorax/respiratory

15 Unknown primary (CUP)

*Enter desired number OR type in a diagnosis and press CR.

> 2

CANCER INFORMATION MENU

BREAST CANCER

Information for Patients   State-of-the-Art Information

                                            4 Prognosis
1 Prognostic Statement   5 Cellular Classification
2 Stage Explanations   6 Stage Information
3 General Treatment Options   7 Treatment by Cell Type/Stage
                        8 Display all information
    9 Continuation options for citation abstracts, CANCERLIT searches and
                                protocols

*Enter desired number and press CR.

> 8

PRINT OPTIONS FOR CANCER INFORMATION

BREAST CANCER

   1 Display all Information for Patients (1–3)
   2 Display all State-of-the-Art Information (4–7)
   3 Display all Information (1–7)
   4 Return to the Cancer Information Menu

*Enter desired number and press CR.

> 2

Breast cancer

Breast cancer is highly treatable using current modalities of surgery, radiation therapy, chemotherapy, and hormonal therapy. Breast cancer is most often curable when detected in early stages. The prognosis and the selection of therapy are influenced by the stage of the disease, pathologic characteristics of the primary tumor, the estrogen and progesterone receptor level in the tumor tissue, measures of proliferative capacity, the age, menopausal status, and general health of the patient. Since criteria of menopausal status vary widely, age greater than 50 can be substituted as a definition of the postmenopausal state. Breast cancer is classified into a variety of cell types, but only a few of these affect prognosis or selection of therapy. Rarely, the breast may be involved by other tumors such as melanoma or lymphoma.

The approach to this disease generally includes a sequence of detection and confirmation of diagnosis, evaluation of stage of disease, and selection of therapy. The confirmation of diagnosis may be by aspiration cytology, needle biopsy, or incisional or excisional biopsy. At the time of surgical removal of tumor tissue, part of the tissue should be processed for determination of estrogen and progesterone receptor levels. This involves either immediate freezing at −70 degrees C and storage at −70 degrees C until assayed, or immediate processing by the laboratory. The assay procedure is technically demanding, and the laboratory should use appropriate quality control procedures. [ref: 2]

Although anatomic stage (axillary node status, size of primary tumor) remains an important prognostic factor, there has been considerable progress made in the identification of other histologic and biologic characteristics that have predictive value. Studies from the National Surgical Adjuvant Breast and Bowel Project (NSABP) and the Ludwig Breast Cancer Study Group have shown that tumor nuclear grade and histologic tumor grade respectively are significant indicators of outcome following adjuvant therapy for breast cancer. However, it is not clear how effectively these pathological factors can be applied outside of these study groups. There is substantial evidence that estrogen receptor status and measures of proliferative capacity of the primary tumor (thymidine labeling index or flow cytometric measurements of S-phase and ploidy) have significant predictive value for patients with stage I disease. In stage II disease, the progesterone receptor status may have greater prognostic value than the estrogen receptor. [ref: 3,4,5,6,7]

Breast cancer is a multicentric disease. However, the occurrence of two or more clinically overt primary cancers in a single breast is uncommon. Likewise, the incidence of a second primary of clinical significance in the opposite breast is uncommon. Synchronous, bilateral cancer is uncommon. Patients who have breast cancer should have bilateral mammography at the time of diagnosis to rule out synchronous disease and should continue to have regular breast physical examinations and mammography to detect asynchronous disease in any remaining breast tissue. Life-long follow-up is required to detect recurrences which can occur as late as 30 years after the initial diagnosis. [ref: 8]

Even when standard therapy is effective, patients with breast cancer are appropriately considered as candidates in clinical trials designed to improve therapeutic results and decrease the morbidity of treatment.
References:

1. Cascinelli N, Greco M, Bufalino R, et al.: Prognosis of breast cancer with axillary node metastases after surgical treatment only.
   European Journal of Cancer and Clinical Oncology 23(6): 795–799, 1987
2. Fisher B, Fisher ER, Redmond C, et al.: Tumor nuclear grade, estrogen receptor, and progesterone receptor: their value alone or in combination as indicators of outcome following adjuvant therapy for breast cancer.
   Breast Cancer Research and Treatment 7(3): 147–160, 1986
3. Davis BW, Gelber RD, Goldhirsch A, et al.: Prognostic significance of tumor grade in clinical trials of adjuvant therapy for breast cancer with axillary lymph node metastasis.
   Cancer 58(12): 2662–2670, 1986
4. Silvestrini R, Daidone MG, Di Fronzo G, et al.: Prognostic implication of labeling index versus estrogen receptors and tumor size in node-negative breast cancer.
   Breast Cancer Research and Treatment 7(3): 161–169, 1986
5. Coulson PB, Thornthwaite JT, Woolley TW, et al.: Prognostic indicators including DNA histogram type, receptor content, and staging related to human breast cancer patient survival.
   Cancer Research 44(9): 4187–4196, 1984
6. McGuire WL, Clark GM, Dressler LG, et al.: Role of steroid hormone receptors as prognostic factors in primary breast cancer.
   National Cancer Institute Monographs 1: 19–23, 1986
7. Moot SK, Peters GN, Cheek JH: Tumor hormone receptor status and

recurrences in premenopausal node negative breast carcinoma.
Cancer 60(3): 382–385, 1987
8. Fisher ER, Fisher B, Sass R, et al.: Pathologic findings from the
National Surgical Adjuvant Breast Project (protocol no. 4): XI.
Bilateral breast cancer.
Cancer 54(12): 3002–3011, 1984

CELLULAR CLASSIFICATION   01/27/88

Breast cancer

Infiltrating or invasive ductal cancer is the most common cell type
comprising 70–80% of all cases.

ductal
    intraductal (in situ)
    invasive with predominant intraductal component
    invasive, NOS (not otherwise specified)
    comedo
    inflammatory*
    medullary with lymphocytic infiltrate
    mucinous (colloid)
    papillary
    scirrhous
    tubular
    other
lobular**
    in situ
    invasive with predominant in situ component
    invasive
nipple
    Paget's disease, NOS (not otherwise specified)
    Paget's disease with intraductal carcinoma
    Paget's disease with invasive ductal carcinoma
other

*Inflammatory carcinoma is a clinicopathologic entity characterized by
diffuse brawny induration of the skin of the breast with an erysipeloid
edge, usually without an underlying palpable mass. Histologically
inflammatory mammary carcinoma diffusely permeates subdermal
lymphatics. (Inflamed cancers that are clinically similar to the above owing

to inflammation, infection, or necrosis but lack microscopic dermal and subdermal lymphatic involvement are not classified as inflammatory carcinoma.) Most patients with inflammatory breast carcinoma have signs of advanced disease such as palpable nodes or distant metastases at diagnosis. All patients with inflammatory breast carcinoma are managed as patients with stage IIIB or IV disease.

**Lobular carcinoma frequently involves both breasts.

References:

1. Manual for Staging of Cancer
   American Joint Committee on Cancer
   Philadelphia: JB Lippincott Company, 2nd ed., 1983
      Part II: Staging of cancer at specific anatomic sites
      pp 23–243
         Ch 21: Breast
         pp 127–133

STAGING INFORMATION   01/27/88

Breast cancer

This staging system provides a strategy for grouping patients as to prognosis. Therapeutic decisions are formulated in part according to staging categories but primarily on lymph node status, estrogen and progesterone receptor levels in the tumor tissue, menopausal status, and the general health of the patient.

Stages are defined by TNM classification.

—TNM definitions—

Primary tumor (T)

TX: Minimum requirements to assess primary tumor cannot be met

TO: No evidence of primary tumor

Tis: In situ cancer (in situ lobular, pure intraductal, and Paget's disease of the nipple without palpable tumor)

Note 1: Paget's disease with a demonstrable tumor is classified according to size of the tumor.

Note 2: Inflammatory carcinoma should be reported separately.

T1: Tumor 2 cm or less in greatest dimension**

T1a: No fixation to underlying pectoral fascia or muscle

T1b: Fixation to underlying pectoral fascia or muscle

T2: Tumor more than 2 cm but not more than 5 cm in its greatest
   dimension**
   T2a: No fixation to underlying pectoral fascia or muscle
   T2b: Fixation to underlying pectoral fascia or muscle
T3: Tumor more than 5 cm in its greatest dimension**
   T3a: No fixation to underlying pectoral fascia or muscle
   T3b: Fixation to underlying pectoral fascia or muscle
T4: Tumor of any size with direct extension to chest wall or skin
   Note: Chest wall includes ribs, intercostal muscles, and serratus
      anterior muscle, but not pectoral muscle.
   T4a: Fixation to chest wall
   T4b: Edema (including peau d'orange), ulceration of the skin of the
      breast, or satellite skin nodules confined to the same breast
   T4c: Both of the above
   T4d: Inflammatory carcinoma

**Dimpling of the skin, nipple retraction, or other skin changes except
   those in T4b may occur in T1, T2, or T3 without changing the
   classification.

Nodal involvement (N): clinical-diagnostic stage
   NX: Regional lymph nodes cannot be assessed clinically
   N0: Homolateral axillary lymph nodes not considered to contain
      growth
   N1: Movable homolateral axillary nodes considered to contain growth
   N2: Homolateral axillary nodes considered to contain growth and
      fixed to one another or to other structures
   N3: Homolateral supraclavicular or infraclavicular nodes considered to
      contain growth or edema of the arm. (Edema of the arm may be
      caused by lymphatic obstruction, and lymph nodes may not then
      be palpable.)
Nodal Involvement (N): Surgical-evaluative and postsurgical
                        resection-pathologic stage
   NX: Regional lymph nodes cannot be assessed (not removed for study
      or previously removed)
   N0: No evidence of homolateral axillary lymph node metastasis
   N1: Metastasis to movable, homolateral axillary nodes not fixed to
      one another or to other structure
      N1a: Micrometastasis less than 0.2 cm in lymph node(s)
      N1b: Gross metastasis in lymph node(s)
   i: Metastasis more than 0.2 cm but less than 2.0 cm in one to three
      lymph nodes

ii: Metastasis more than 0.2 cm but less than 2.0 cm in four or more lymph nodes

iii: Extension of metastasis beyond the lymph node capsule (less than 2.0 cm in dimension)

iv: Metastasis in lymph node 2.0 cm or more in dimension

    N2: Metastases to homolateral axillary lymph nodes that are fixed to one another or to other structures

    N3: Metastasis to homolateral supraclavicular or infraclavicular lymph node(s)

Note: Edema of the arm may be caused by lymphatic obstruction, and lymph nodes may not then be palpable. Homolateral internal mammary nodes considered to contain growth are included in N3 for surgical-evaluative classification and postsurgical resection-pathologic classification.

Distant metastasis (M)

    MX: Minimum requirements to assess the presence of distant metastasis cannot be met

    M0: No (known) distant metastasis

    M1: Distant metastasis present

    Specify sites according to the following notations:

    PUL   pulmonary
    OSS   osseous
    HEP   hepatic
    BRA   brain
    LYM   lymph nodes
    MAR   bone marrow
    PLE   pleura
    SKI   skin
    EYE   eye
    OTH   other

—In situ—   5-year survival: $>95\%$

In situ breast cancer is defined as the following TNM grouping:

Tis, N0, M0

—Stage I—   5-year survival: 85%

Stage I breast cancer is defined as the following TNM grouping:

T1, N0, M0

—Stage II—   5-year survival: 66%
Stage II breast cancer is defined as any of the following TNM groupings:

> T2, N0, M0
> T0–T2, N1, M0

—Stage III—   5-year survival: 41%
Stage IIIA breast cancer is defined as any of the following TNM groupings:

> T0–T2, N2, M0
> T3, N0–N2, M0

Stage IIIB breast cancer is defined as any of the following TNM groupings:

any T, N3, M0
T4, any N, M0

Note: Inflammatory breast cancer is included in either stage IIIB or stage
      IV, depending on whether metastases are present or not.

—Stage IV—   5-year survival: 10%
Stage IV breast cancer is defined as the following TNM grouping:

any T, any N, M1

Note: Inflammatory breast cancer is included in either stage IIIB or stage
      IV, depending on whether metastases are present or not.
References:
1. Manual for Staging of Cancer
   American Joint Committee on Cancer
   Philadelphia: JB Lippincott Company, 2nd ed., 1983
      Part II: Staging of cancer at specific anatomic sites
      pp 23–243
         Ch 21: Breast
         pp 127–133

TREATMENT OVERVIEW   01/27/88

Breast cancer

State-of-the-art treatment in breast cancer is influenced by the stage,
hormone receptor levels, age, and menopausal status. All newly
diagnosed patients with breast cancer may appropriately be considered

as candidates for one of the numerous ongoing clinical trials designed to improve survival and decrease the morbidity of current treatment.

TREATMENT BY CELL TYPE OR STAGE   01/27/88

Breast cancer in situ

Noninvasive cancers constitute 5 to 10 percent of breast cancers. Such cancers are classified as lobular carcinoma in situ arising from the epithelium of the lobules or intraductal arising from ductal epithelium. Both types of in situ carcinoma are curable. [ref: 1]

The customary treatment for noninvasive intraductal cancers has been mastectomy with a simultaneous low axillary dissection. The role of breast conserving operations for noninvasive intraductal carcinoma is the subject of ongoing prospective randomized clinical trials. Limited experience with conservative surgery and radiation therapy suggests that local control with this approach is acceptable and overall survival excellent. If margins of the initial excisional biopsy are positive or questionable, reexcision should be done prior to beginning radiation therapy. A simultaneous low axillary dissection is not mandatory as positive lymph nodes are rare. Those patients in whom lymph node involvement is documented should be managed as described under stage II.

Because of the risk of invasive cancer developing in either breast in a patient with lobular carcinoma in situ, the treatment options range from excisional biopsy plus observation to bilateral total mastectomies. The incidence of axillary metastases is low, but low axillary sampling is often performed.

Reconstructive surgery:
For breast cancer in situ, stage I, and stage II, reconstructive surgery may be employed if a mastectomy is performed. It may be done at the time of the mastectomy (immediate reconstruction) or at some subsequent time (delayed reconstruction), in an attempt to restore the anatomical deficit of the mastectomy. [ref: 2,3,4]

Treatment options for intraductal carcinoma: [ref: 5]

Standard:

1. Segmental/wedge/partial breast resection with or without simultaneous low axillary dissection.

2. Excisional biopsy with radiation therapy with or without simultaneous low axillary dissection.
3. Total mastectomy with or without low axillary dissection.

Treatment options for lobular carcinoma in situ: [ref: 6]

Standard:

1. Excisional biopsy with or without low axillary dissection.
2. Unilateral total mastectomy with or without low axillary dissection.
3. Bilateral total mastectomies with or without low axillary dissection.

References:

1. Breast Cancer—Diagnosis and Treatment
   Ariel IM, Cleary JB, Eds.
   New York: McGraw-Hill, 1987
   Ch 16: The management of clinically nonpalpable breast cancer
   Leis HP, Cammarata A, LaRaja RD
   pp 205–223
2. Feller WF, Holt R, Spear S, et al.: Modified radical mastectomy with immediate breast reconstruction.
   American Surgeon 52(3): 129–133, 1986
3. Woods JE: Breast reconstruction: current state of the art.
   Mayo Clinic Proceedings 61(7): 579–585, 1986
4. Advances in Breast and Endocrine Surgery
   Najarian JS, Delaney JP, Eds.
   Chicago: Year Book Medical Publishers, 1986
     Breast reconstruction following mastectomy
     Cunningham BL
     pp 213–226
5. Secht A, Danoff BS, Solin LJ, et al.: Intraductal carcinoma of the breast: results of treatment with excisional biopsy and irradiation.
   Journal of Clinical Oncology 3(10): 1339–1343, 1985
6. Hutter RV: The management of patients with lobular carcinoma in situ of the breast.
   Cancer 53(Suppl 3): 798–802, 1984

Stage I breast cancer

Stage I breast cancer is highly curable with a range of surgical procedures. Surgical procedures which conserve a major portion of the involved breast, followed by radiotherapy, provides tumor control equivalent to more extensive surgical procedures. The diagnostic biopsy and the surgical procedure that will be used as primary treatment should be performed as two separate procedures. After the presence of a malignancy is confirmed, and the histology is determined, treatment options should be discussed with the patient before definitive therapy is recommended. Estrogen and progesterone receptor proteins should be determined for the primary tumor. [ref: 1]

In many cases, the diagnosis of breast carcinoma using fine needle aspiration cytology may be sufficient to confirm malignancy. It is then appropriate to discuss the therapeutic options of mastectomy versus conservative surgery and radiation therapy to help the patient with the treatment decision. The surgeon may then proceed with biopsy, frozen section confirmation of carcinoma, followed by the definitive local procedure elected by the patient as a single procedure.

Selection of the appropriate therapeutic approach depends on the location and size of the lesion, breast size, and whether the patient feels strongly about preservation of the breast. Postoperative chest wall radiation therapy after modified or total mastectomy should not be given routinely and should only be performed in selected patients who are known to have residual tumor in the operative field or may be in the high-risk groups for local/regional failure. An axillary node dissection should be performed for histologic study since approximately one-third of patients with clinically negative nodes will have histologic involvement and may be candidates for additional treatment as per stage II (axillary nodes involved). In addition, estrogen receptor status, tumor size, and measures of proliferative capacity (thymidine labeling index, flow cytometry for measurement of S-phase and ploidy) are highly predictive for risk of relapse in the node-negative patient. [ref: 2]

Reconstructive surgery:
For breast cancer in situ, stage I, and stage II, reconstructive surgery may be employed if a mastectomy is performed. It may be done at the time of the mastectomy (immediate reconstruction) or at some subsequent time (delayed reconstruction), in an attempt to restore the anatomical deficit of the mastectomy. [ref: 3,4,5]

Treatment options:

Standard:
One of the following surgical procedures, listed in the order of limited to extensive, is used for initial treatment depending on the location and size of the lesion, breast size, and whether the patient feels strongly about preservation of the breast. The first two procedures are appropriate when

negative margins can be achieved at the time of excision. If one of the first two procedures is performed, radiotherapy is used to treat the remaining breast tissue. Treatment consists of external beam radiation therapy plus an optional boost of interstitial radioactive implants (or an optional booster dose of external radiation) to the primary tumor site. The primary advantage of this approach for the patient is cosmesis. Surgical and radiotherapeutic technique are extremely important in obtaining an optimal therapeutic result and satisfactory cosmesis. The availability of specialized equipment and radiotherapists with expertise using this approach should be considered in the selection of treatment.

1. Excisional biopsy/lumpectomy with separate axillary node dissection and radiotherapy to breast. [ref: 6,7,8,9,10,11,12]
2. Segmental/wedge/partial breast resection with axillary node dissection and radiotherapy to breast. [ref: 6,7,8,10]
3. Modified radical or total mastectomy with axillary dissection. [ref: 6,13,14]

Investigational:
Following surgery or limited surgery and radiotherapy, investigational protocols exploring the value of adjuvant chemotherapy or hormonal therapy for patients with negative nodes, but poor prognostic features of the primary tumor, should be considered. Such features include absence of hormone receptors, large tumor size, poorly differentiated pathology, and high proliferative capacity. For good prognosis node-negative patients with positive estrogen receptors, an NSABP trial randomizes patients between tamoxifen and placebo. [ref: 15]

References:

1. Fisher B, Fisher ER, Redmond C, et al.: Tumor nuclear grade, estrogen receptor, and progesterone receptor: their value alone or in combination as indicators of outcome following adjuvant therapy for breast cancer.
   Breast Cancer Research and Treatment 7(3): 147–160, 1986
2. Meyer JS: Cell kinetics in selection and stratification of patients for adjuvant therapy of breast carcinoma.
   National Cancer Institute Monographs 1: 25–28, 1986
3. Feller WF, Holt R, Spear S, et al.: Modified radical mastectomy with immediate breast reconstruction.
   American Surgeon 52(3): 129–133, 1986
4. Woods JE: Breast reconstruction: current state of the art.
   Mayo Clinic Proceedings 61(7): 579–585, 1986

5. Advances in Breast and Endocrine Surgery
   Najarian JS, Delaney JP, Eds.
   Chicago: Year Book Medical Publishers, 1986
      Breast reconstruction following mastectomy
      Cunningham BL
      pp 213–226

6. Veronesi U, Saccozzi R, Del Vecchio M, et al.: Comparing radical mastectomy with quadrantectomy, axillary dissection, and radiotherapy in patients with small cancers of the breast.
   New England Journal of Medicine 305(1): 6–11, 1981

7. Levene MB, Harris JR, Hellman S: Treatment of carcinoma of the breast by radiation therapy.
   Cancer 39(6): 2840–2845, 1977

8. Romsdahl MM, Montague ED, Ames FC, et al.: Conservative surgery and irradiation as treatment for early breast cancer.
   Archives of Surgery 118(5): 521–526, 1983

9. Fisher B, Bauer M, Margolese R, et al.: Five-year results of a randomized clinical trial comparing total mastectomy and segmental mastectomy with or without radiation in the treatment of breast cancer.
   New England Journal of Medicine 312(12): 665–673, 1985

10. Veronesi U, Zucali R, Luini A: Local control and survival in early breast cancer: the Milan trial.
    International Journal of Radiation Oncology, Biology, Physics 12(5): 717–720, 1986

11. Veronesi U, Banfi A, Del Vecchio M, et al.: Comparison of Halsted mastectomy with quadrantectomy, axillary dissection, and radiotherapy in early breast cancer: long-term results.
    European Journal of Cancer and Clinical Oncology 22(9): 1085–1089, 1986

12. Kurtz JM, Amalric R, DeLouche G, et al.: The second ten years: Long-term risks of breast conservation in early breast cancer.
    International Journal of Radiation Oncology, Biology, Physics 13(9): 1327–1332, 1987

13. Fisher B, Redmond C, Fisher ER, et al.: Ten-year results of a randomized clinical trial comparing radical mastectomy and total mastectomy with or without radiation.
    New England Journal of Medicine 312(11): 674–681, 1985

14. Martin JK, van Heerden JA, Taylor WF, et al.: Is modified radical mastectomy really equivalent to radical mastectomy in treatment of carcinoma of the breast?
Cancer 57(3): 510–518, 1986
15. National Institutes of Health Consensus Development Conference statement: adjuvant chemotherapy for breast cancer.
Journal of the American Medical Association 254(24): 3461–3463, 1985

Stage II breast cancer

Stage II breast cancer is curable with a range of accepted surgical procedures. Conservative surgical approaches which salvage a portion of the breast followed by postoperative radiation therapy can provide tumor control equivalent to more extensive surgery. The diagnostic biopsy and the surgical procedure that will be used as primary treatment should be performed as two separate procedures. After the presence of a malignancy is confirmed, and the histology is determined, treatment options should be discussed with the patient before a definitive therapeutic procedure is recommended. Estrogen and progesterone receptor proteins should be determined on the primary tumor. [ref: 1]

In many cases, the diagnosis of breast carcinoma using fine needle aspiration cytology may be sufficient to confirm malignancy. It is then appropriate to discuss the therapeutic options of mastectomy versus conservative surgery and radiation therapy to help the patient with the treatment decision. The surgeon may then proceed with biopsy, frozen section confirmation of carcinoma, followed by the definitive local procedure elected by the patient as a single procedure.

Selection of one of the equivalent treatment options depends on the location and size of the lesion, breast size, and whether the patient feels strongly about preservation of the breast. Postoperative chest wall radiation therapy after modified radical or total mastectomy is not given routinely and should only be recommended for highly selected patients who are known to have residual tumor left in the operative field, or are at high risk for microscopic residual disease including patients with more than 4 positive axillary lymph nodes or if there is lymphatic permeation in the breast. An axillary dissection should be done for histologic study. Adjuvant combination chemotherapy has been found to prolong disease-free interval and survival for premenopausal patients with positive nodes. The standard duration of administration of such chemotherapy does not exceed one year. For node positive postmenopausal women with hormone positive receptor tumors, adjuvant hormonal therapy with the relatively nontoxic anti-estrogen tamoxifen prolongs disease-free interval and perhaps survival. In this setting, tamoxifen should be given for at least two years. Adjuvant combination chemotherapy has more modest, but probably significant, survival impact in node positive postmenopausal women. For some postmenopausal patients with negative hormone receptors, these small advantages may outweigh the toxicity of chemotherapy. The role of adjuvant chemotherapy/hormonal therapy for node negative patients is under investigation. All newly diagnosed patients with breast cancer can, if circumstances permit, be appropriately referred to one of the many clinical trials in progress to evaluate new treatments and improve older approaches (see investigative protocols). [ref: 2,3]

Dose intensity:

Recent retrospective analyses have indicated that the intensity of dose delivery may be important in the clinical outcome. Dose intensity is expressed in mg/m2 per week. Analyses of trials using a combination of drugs have, in general, given equal weighting to the "effective drugs" and have assigned a zero value if a given "standard" drug is not used in a particular regimen. Therefore, there is some degree of subjectivity to these analyses. Nevertheless, using such analyses, response rate (in advanced breast cancer) and freedom from relapse (in stage II breast cancer) have increased with increasing dose intensity. The steepest relationship between dose intensity and outcome has come from dose intensities of less than 0.8. Physicians should avoid arbitrary reductions in dose intensity. [ref: 4,5,6]

Reconstructive surgery:

For breast cancer in situ, stage I, and stage II, reconstructive surgery may be employed if a mastectomy is performed. It may be done at the time of the mastectomy (immediate reconstruction) or at some subsequent time (delayed reconstruction), in an attempt to restore the anatomical deficit of the mastectomy. [ref: 7,8,9]

Treatment options:

Standard:

1. One of the following surgical procedures, listed in the order of limited to extensive is used for initial treatment depending on the location and size of the lesion, breast size, and whether the patient feels strongly about preservation of the breast. The first two procedures are appropriate for primary tumors less than or equal to

4 cm in size and when negative margins can be achieved at the time of excision. If one of the first two procedures is performed, radiotherapy is used to treat the remaining breast tissue. Treatment consists of external beam radiation plus an optional boost of interstitial radioactive implants (or an optional booster dose of external radiation) to the primary tumor site. The primary advantage of this approach for the patient is cosmesis. Surgical and radiotherapeutic technique are extremely important in obtaining an optimal therapeutic result and satisfactory cosmesis. The availability of specialized equipment and radiotherapists with expertise using this approach should be considered in the selection of treatment. The surgical procedures include:

excisional biopsy/lumpectomy with separate axillary node dissection and radiotherapy to breast [ref: 10,11,12,13,14,15,16]

segmental/wedge/partial breast resection with axillary node dissection and radiotherapy to breast [ref: 10,11,12,14]

modified radical or total mastectomy [ref: 10,17,18]

radical mastectomy (in selected circumstances only, if needed to accomplish complete tumor resection)

2. Following the treatment used to control local disease, adjuvant combination chemotherapy is given to reduce the rate of recurrence and improve survival in premenopausal patients with lymph node involvement. Many different drug regimens have been developed. Numerous studies have shown that combination chemotherapy is superior to single-agent treatment, and single-agent adjuvant chemotherapy should be avoided outside a clinical trial. The drug combinations listed have been tested and provide therapeutic benefit. Not all have been compared to an untreated control group in prospective randomized trials.

CMF: cyclophosphamide + methotrexate + fluorouracil [ref: 19,20]

CMFVP: cyclophosphamide + methotrexate + fluorouracil + vincristine + prednisone [ref: 21]

L-PAM and 5-FU: melphalan + fluorouracil, for premenopausal women [ref: 22,23]

L-PAM, 5-FU, and tamoxifen: melphalan + fluorouracil + tamoxifen, for postmenopausal women whose tumors are estrogen/progesterone receptor positive [ref: 24]

CA: cyclophosphamide + doxorubicin* [ref: 25]

CAF: cytoxan + doxorubicin* + fluorouracil [ref: 26]

*The potential for doxorubicin-induced cardiotoxicity should be considered in the selection of chemotherapeutic regimens for an individual patient.

3. Following the treatment used to control local disease, adjuvant endocrine therapy with tamoxifen alone is given to reduce the rate of recurrence and probably improve survival in postmenopausal patients with lymph node involvement and positive hormone receptors. Tamoxifen, either alone or combined with chemotherapy, prolongs disease-free survival when administered for 24 months as adjuvant therapy to postmenopausal women with axillary lymph node metastases. It is probably of additional benefit when given for an even longer period of time. [ref: 3,27,28,29,30]

Investigational:

Investigational protocols evaluating new types of chemotherapy and/or hormone therapy.

While significant advances have been made in the past five years, optimal adjuvant therapy has not been defined for any subset of patients. For this reason, all patients and their physicians are strongly encouraged to participate in controlled clinical trials. [ref: 27]

References:

1. Fisher B, Fisher ER, Redmond C, et al.: Tumor nuclear grade, estrogen receptor, and progesterone receptor: their value alone or in combination as indicators of outcome following adjuvant therapy for breast cancer.
Breast Cancer Research and Treatment 7(3): 147–160, 1986
2. Review of mortality results in randomized trials in early breast cancer.
Lancet 2(8413): 1205, 1984
3. Baum M, Brinkley DM, Dossett JA, et al.: Controlled trial of tamoxifen as single adjuvant agent in management of early breast cancer: analysis at six years by Nolvadex Adjuvant Trial Organization.
Lancet 1(8433): 836–840, 1985
4. Hryniuk W, Levine MN: Analysis of dose intensity for adjuvant chemotherapy trials in stage II breast cancer.
Journal of Clinical Oncology 4(8): 1162–1170, 1986
5. Hryniuk WM, Levine MN, Levin L: Analysis of dose intensity for chemotherapy in early (stage II) and advanced breast cancer.
National Cancer Institute Monographs 1: 87–94, 1986
6. Hryniuk WM: Average relative dose intensity and the impact on design of clinical trials.
Seminars in Oncology 14(1): 65–74, 1987
7. Feller WF, Holt R, Spear S, et al.: Modified radical mastectomy with immediate breast reconstruction.
American Surgeon 52(3): 129–133, 1986

8. Woods JE: Breast reconstruction: current state of the art.
   Mayo Clinic Proceedings 61(7): 579–585, 1986

9. Advances in Breast and Endocrine Surgery
   Najarian JS, Delaney JP, Eds.
   Chicago: Year Book Medical Publishers, 1986
      Breast reconstruction following mastectomy
      Cunningham BL
      pp 213–226

10. Veronesi U, Saccozzi R, Del Vecchio M, et al.: Comparing radical
    mastectomy with quadrantectomy, axillary dissection, and
    radiotherapy in patients with small cancers of the breast.
    New England Journal of Medicine 305(1): 6–11, 1981

11. Levene MB, Harris JR, Hellman S: Treatment of carcinoma of the
    breast by radiation therapy.
    Cancer 39(6): 2840–2845, 1977

12. Romsdahl MM, Montague ED, Ames FC, et al.: Conservative surgery
    and irradiation as treatment for early breast cancer.
    Archives of Surgery 118(5): 521–526, 1983

13. Fisher B, Bauer M, Margolese R, et al.: Five-year results of a
    randomized clinical trial comparing total mastectomy and segmental
    mastectomy with or without radiation in the treatment of breast
    cancer.
    New England Journal of Medicine 312(12): 665–673, 1985

14. Veronesi U, Zucali R, Luini A: Local control and survival in early
    breast cancer: the Milan trial.
    International Journal of Radiation Oncology, Biology, Physics 12(5):
    717–720, 1986

15. Veronesi U, Banfi A, Del Vecchio M, et al.: Comparison of Halsted
    mastectomy with quadrantectomy, axillary dissection, and
    radiotherapy in early breast cancer: long-term results.
    European Journal of Cancer and Clinical Oncology 22(9):
    1085–1089, 1986

16. Kurtz JM, Amalric R, DeLouche G, et al.: The second ten years:
    Long-term risks of breast conservation in early breast cancer.
    International Journal of Radiation Oncology, Biology, Physics 13(9):
    1327–1332, 1987

17. Fisher B, Redmond C, Fisher ER, et al.: Ten-year results of a
    randomized clinical trial comparing radical mastectomy and total
    mastectomy with or without radiation.
    New England Journal of Medicine 312(11): 674–681, 1985

18. Martin JK, van Heerden JA, Taylor WF, et al.: Is modified radical

mastectomy really equivalent to radical mastectomy in treatment of carcinoma of the breast?
Cancer 57(3): 510–518, 1986

19. Tancini G, Bonadonna G, Valagussa P, et al.: Adjuvant CMF in breast cancer: comparative 5-year results of 12 versus 6 cycles. Journal of Clinical Oncology 1(1): 2–10, 1983

20. Bonadonna G, Brusamolino E, Valagussa P, et al.: Combination chemotherapy as an adjuvant treatment in operable breast cancer. New England Journal of Medicine 294(8): 405–410, 1976

21. Glucksberg H, Rivkin SE, Rasmussen S, et al.: Combination chemotherapy (CMFVP) versus L-phenylalanine mustard (L-PAM) for operable breast cancer with positive axillary nodes: a Southwest Oncology Group study.
Cancer 50(3): 423–434, 1982

22. Fisher ER, Redmond C, Fisher B: Pathologic findings from the National Surgical Adjuvant Breast Project: VIII. Relationship of chemotherapeutic responsiveness to tumor differentiation.
Cancer 51(2): 181–191, 1983

23. Fisher B, Glass A, Redmond C., et al.: L-phenylalanine mustard (L-PAM) in the management of primary breast cancer: an update of earlier findings and a comparison with those utilizing L-PAM plus 5-fluorouracil (5-FU).
Cancer 39(Suppl 6): 2883–2903, 1977

24. Fisher B, Redmond C, Brown A, et al.: Adjuvant chemotherapy with and without tamoxifen in the treatment of primary breast cancer: 5-year results from the National Surgical Adjuvant Breast and Bowel Project Clinical Trial.
Journal of Clinical Oncology 4(4): 459–471, 1986

25. Jones SE, Salmon SE, Allen H, et al.: Adjuvant treatment of node-positive breast cancer with Adriamycin-cyclophosphamide with or without radiation therapy: interim results of an ongoing clinical trial.
Recent Results in Cancer Research 80: 162–169, 1982

26. Buzdar AU, Blumenschein GR, Smith TL, et al.: Adjuvant chemotherapy with fluorouracil, doxorubicin, and cyclophosphamide, with or without bacillus Calmette-Guerin and with or without irradiation in operable breast cancer.
Cancer 53(3): 384–389, 1984

27. National Institutes of Health Consensus Development Conference statement: adjuvant chemotherapy for breast cancer.

Journal of the American Medical Association 254(24): 3461–3463, 1985

28. Fisher B, Brown A, Wolmark N, et al.: Prolonging tamoxifen therapy for primary breast cancer: findings from the National Surgical Adjuvant Breast and Bowel Project Clinical Trial.
Annals of Internal Medicine 106(5): 649–654, 1987

29. Cummings FJ, Gray R, Davis TE, et al.: Adjuvant tamoxifen treatment of elderly women with stage II breast cancer: a double-blind comparison with placebo.
Annals of Internal Medicine 103(3): 324–329, 1985

30. Bartlett K, Eremin O, Hutcheon A., et al.: Adjuvant tamoxifen in the management of operable breast cancer: The Scottish Trial.
Lancet 2(8552): 171–175, 1987

Stage III breast cancer

Stage III breast cancer is further classified into operable (stage IIIA) and inoperable (locally advanced, stage IIIB) disease. Stage IIIA disease is responsive to therapy, and control of disease for long periods of time is often possible. Treatment plans for stage IIIA breast cancer often include sequential use of surgery, radiation therapy, and chemotherapy.

—Stage IIIA (operable breast cancer)—

Treatment options:

Standard:

1. One of the following surgical procedures for initial treatment:
   modified radical mastectomy
   radical mastectomy
2. Because of the high risk of local recurrence for this stage, radiation therapy should be considered as part of the overall treatment plan:
   preoperative external beam radiation
   postoperative external beam radiation with a booster dose to the primary tumor site
3. Chemotherapy regimens with or without hormones are given in conjunction with the above surgical procedures. Some of the equally effective combination chemotherapy regimens commonly used are:
   CMF: cyclophosphamide + methotrexate + fluorouracil [ref: 2]
   CAF: cyclophosphamide + doxorubicin* + fluorouracil [ref: 3]
   CMFP: cyclophosphamide + methotrexate + fluorouracil + prednisone [ref: 4]

CMFVP: cyclophosphamide + methotrexate + fluorouracil + vincristine + prednisone [ref: 5]

L-PAM and 5-FU: melphalan + fluorouracim, for premenopausal women [ref: 6,7]

L-PAM, 5-FU and tamoxifen: melphalan + fluorouracil + tamoxifen, for postmenopausal women whose tumors are estrogen/progesterone positive [ref: 8]

CA: cyclophosphamide + doxorubicin* [ref: 9]

*The potential for doxorubicin-induced cardiotoxicity should be considered in the selection of chemotherapeutic regimens for an individual patient.

Investigational:

Investigational protocols evaluating the role of combination chemotherapy with or without hormonal manipulation are underway. Tamoxifen as postoperative adjuvant hormonal therapy for postmenopausal patients with high levels of estrogen and progesterone receptors can be given in addition to adjuvant chemotherapy. [ref: 8]

—Stage IIIB (inoperable breast cancer, including inflammatory)—

Radiation therapy has an important role in controlling local and regional disease in patients who present with inoperable stage III disease. Systemic chemotherapy is recommended to control occult metastatic disease. Surgery may be employed for a diagnostic biopsy, or for removal of tumor following other therapy. The sequencing of local therapy versus systemic therapy is under investigation. Treatment plans generally include a combination of surgery (for diagnosis), radiation therapy (pre- or postoperative electron beam therapy), and chemotherapy. Patients should be considered candidates for one of the ongoing clinical trials in progress to improve therapeutic results in this disease.

In stage IIIB breast cancer, surgery is generally limited to the initial biopsy. Radiation therapy is used to treat the local disease and chemotherapy is used to treat occult metastases. For patients with stage III breast cancers, the use of initial chemotherapy after biopsy and prior to local therapy with surgery or radiation therapy may offer advantages of tumor shrinkage and early systemic control. A recent preliminary report observed biopsy confirmed complete responses of breast tumor masses following combination chemotherapy prior to local treatment. Surgical removal of residual tumor may be performed, if a good response is achieved with the other therapies employed. Newly diagnosed patients with stage III breast cancer should be considered candidates for one of the clinical trials in progress to improve therapeutic results in this disease. [ref: 10]

Treatment options:

Standard:

1. Incisional biopsy for diagnosis and receptor protein assay followed by external beam radiation to the primary and to the regional nodes. If the patient has a good response, a cone down field with external beam radiation plus interstitial implants to the primary site may be recommended. If the response is poor, a mastectomy may be performed if technically feasible, or continued radiotherapy with a cone down field may be recommended.
2. After the surgery and radiotherapy described above is completed, one of the following chemotherapy regimens may be considered:
CMF: cyclophosphamide + methotrexate + fluorouracil [ref: 2]
CAF: cyclophosphamide + doxorubicin* + fluorouracil [ref: 3]
CMFP: cyclophosphamide + methotrexate + fluorouracil + prednisone [ref: 11]
CMFVP: cyclophosphamide + methotrexate + fluorouracil + vincristine + prednisone [ref: 5]
CA: cyclophosphamide + doxorubicin* [ref: 9]

*The potential for doxorubicin-induced cardiotoxicity should be considered in the selection of chemotherapeutic regimens for an individual patient.

3. If combination chemotherapy is contraindicated, one of the following hormonal therapies may be recommended for patients whose tumors are positive for estrogen and progesterone receptor proteins after the surgery and radiotherapy described above is completed:
oophorectomy for premenopausal patients
tamoxifen for postmenopausal patients [ref: 8]
estrogen for postmenopausal patients
progesterone therapy
androgen for pre- or postmenopausal patients

Investigational:

1. Studies utilizing combination chemotherapy initially followed by surgery and/or radiation therapy, and maintenance chemotherapy have been instituted. [ref: 12]

2. Phase II studies evaluating newly developed chemotherapeutic agents or biologicals may also be considered for patients whose local disease is not controllable by standard measures.

References:

1. Perry MC, Kardinal CG, Korzun AH, et al.: Chemohormonal therapy in advanced carcinoma of the breast: Cancer and Leukemia Group B protocol 8081.
   Journal of Clinical Oncology 5(10): 1534–1545, 1987
2. Tancini G, Bonadonna G, Valagussa P, et al.: Adjuvant CMF in breast cancer: comparative 5-year results of 12 versus 6 cycles.
   Journal of Clinical Oncology 1(1): 2–10, 1983
3. Buzdar AU, Smith TL, Powell KC, et al.: Effect of timing of initiation of adjuvant chemotherapy on disease-free survival in breast cancer.
   Breast Cancer Research and Treatment 2(2): 163–169, 1982
4. Adjuvant Therapy of Cancer IV
   Jones SE, Salmon SE, Eds.
   New York: Grune and Stratton, Inc., 1984
     A summary of findings from NSABP: trials of adjuvant therapy
     Fisher B, Redmond C, Fisher ER, et al.
     pp 185–194
5. Glucksberg H, Rivkin SE, Rasmussen S, et al.: Combination chemotherapy (CMFVP) versus L-phenylalanine mustard (L-PAM) for operable breast cancer with positive axillary nodes: a Southwest Oncology Group study.
   Cancer 50(3): 423–434, 1982
6. Fisher ER, Redmond C, Fisher B: Pathologic findings from the National Surgical Adjuvant Breast Project: VIII. Relationship of chemotherapeutic responsiveness to tumor differentiation.
   Cancer 51(2): 181–191, 1983
7. Fisher B, Glass A, Redmond C., et al.: L-phenylalanine mustard (L-PAM) in the management of primary breast cancer: an update of earlier findings and a comparison with those utilizing L-PAM plus 5-fluorouracil (5-FU).
   Cancer 39(Suppl 6): 2883–2903, 1977
8. Fisher B, Redmond C, Brown A, et al.: Influence of tumor estrogen and progesterone receptor levels on the response to tamoxifen and chemotherapy in primary breast cancer.
   Journal of Clinical Oncology 1(4): 227–241, 1983
9. Jones SE, Salmon SE, Allen H, et al.: Adjuvant treatment of node-positive breast cancer with Adriamycin-cyclophosphamide with

or without radiation therapy: interim results of an ongoing clinical trial.
Recent Results in Cancer Research 80: 162–169, 1982

10. Swain SM, Sorace RA, Bagley CS, et al.: Neoadjuvant chemotherapy in the combined modality approach of locally advanced nonmetastatic breast cancer
Cancer Research 47(14): 3889–3894, 1987

11. Tormey DC, Gelman R, Band PR, et al.: Comparison of induction chemotherapies for metastatic breast cancer: an Eastern Cooperative Oncology Group trial.
Cancer 50(7): 1235–1244, 1982

12. Hortobagyi GN, Blumenschein GR, Spanos W, et al.: Multimodal treatment of locoregionally advanced breast cancer.
Cancer 51(5): 763–768, 1983

Stage IV breast cancer

Stage IV breast cancer is often responsive to treatment with durable complete remissions attainable in 10–20% of patients, although long disease-free survival compatible with cure is rare. Surgical procedures are generally limited to those that will permit the determination of histology and estrogen and progesterone receptor levels. Control of local disease is achieved with either surgery or radiotherapy. External beam radiation also has a major role in the palliation of symptoms, particularly pain caused by bone metastases. All patients with stage IV breast cancer should be considered candidates for one of the ongoing clinical trials in progress to improve therapeutic results in this disease. The treatment of inflammatory breast cancer and stage IV breast cancer is similar.

Treatment options:

Standard:

1. A surgical biopsy to determine histology and estrogen and progesterone receptor levels. External beam radiotherapy or a hygienic mastectomy may be recommended to control local disease.

2. If visceral disease is absent and estrogen and progesterone receptor status is positive, hormonal therapy is an excellent first treatment. One of the following equivalent approaches can be used:
tamoxifen or oophorectomy for premenopausal patients [ref: 2]
antiestrogen therapy with tamoxifen for postmenopausal patients
estrogen therapy for postmenopausal patients
progestational agents for postmenopausal agents

3. If visceral disease is present or estrogen and progesterone receptor status is negative, one of the following combination chemotherapy regimens will produce equivalent results:
   CMF: cyclophosphamide + methotrexate + fluorouracil [ref: 3]
   CAF: cyclophosphamide + doxorubicin* + fluorouracil [ref: 4]
   CMFP: cyclophosphamide + methotrexate + fluorouracil + prednisone [ref: 3]
   CMFVP: cyclophosphamide + methotrexate + fluorouracil + vincristine + prednisone [ref: 4]
   CA: cyclophosphamide + doxorubicin* [ref: 5]

*The potential for doxorubicin-induced cardiotoxicity should be considered in the selection of chemotherapeutic regimens for an individual patient.

Investigational:

1. If visceral disease is absent and estrogen and progesterone receptor status is positive, investigational protocols evaluating the role of hormonal therapy should be considered as first treatment.
2. If visceral disease is present or estrogen and progesterone receptor status is negative, investigational protocols evaluating the role of combination chemotherapy with and without hormonal therapy should be considered as first treatment.
3. Phase II studies evaluating newly developed chemotherapeutic agents or biologicals should also be considered.

References:

1. Perry MC, Kardinal CG, Korzun AH, et al.: Chemohormonal therapy in advanced carcinoma of the breast: Cancer and Leukemia Group B protocol 8081.
   Journal of Clinical Oncology 5(10): 1534–1545, 1987
2. Ingle JN, Krook JE, Green SJ, et al.: Randomized trial of bilateral oophorectomy versus tamoxifen in premenopausal women with metastatic breast cancer.
   Journal of Clinical Oncology 4(2): 178–185, 1986
3. Wormey DC, Gelman R, Band PR, et al.: Comparison of induction chemotherapies for metastatic breast cancer: an Eastern Cooperative Oncology Group trial.
   Cancer 50(7): 1235–1244, 1982
4. Smalley RV, Lefante J, Bartolucci A, et al.: A comparison of

cyclophosphamide, Adriamycin, and 5-fluorouracil (CAF) and
cyclophosphamide, methotrexate, 5-fluorouracil, vincristine and
prednisone (CMFVP) in patients with advanced breast cancer: a
Southeastern Cancer Study Group project.
Breast Cancer Research and Treatment 3(2): 209–220, 1983
5. Tranum BL, McDonald B, Thigpen T, et al.: Adriamycin combinations
in advanced breast cancer: a Southwest Oncology Group study.
Cancer 49(5): 835–839, 1982

Recurrent breast cancer

Recurrent breast cancer is often responsive to therapy although treatment
rarely cures this stage of the disease. Radiation therapy has a major role
in the palliation of locally recurrent disease and symptoms such as pain
due to bone metastases. The level of estrogen and progesterone receptor
proteins at the time of recurrence and previous treatment should be used
in selecting therapy. If the estrogen and progesterone receptor status is
unknown or positive, then the site(s) of recurrence, disease-free interval,
response to previous treatment, and menopausal status are useful in
selecting chemotherapy or hormonal therapy. Local recurrence is usually
the harbinger of widespread disease but, in a small subset of patients,
may be the only site of recurrence. For patients in this subset, surgery
and/or radiation therapy may infrequently be curative. [ref: 2]

Approximately one-quarter to one-third of patients with a chest-wall
recurrence following mastectomy will have had preceding distant
metastases. Another one-quarter of patients will develop distant
metastases within a few months of the discovery of local recurrence.
Despite aggressive local treatment with radiotherapy, almost all patients
with even an "isolated" local recurrence will eventually develop distant
metastases. The 5-year disease-free survival rate (i.e. neither further local
or distant relapse) in one recent series of such patients was 30%, with a
10-year rate of 7%. The prognosis following breast recurrence after
conservative surgery and radiation therapy is, however, much better than
that following chest-wall recurrence after mastectomy. Between 9–25% of
such individuals will be found to have distant metastases or locally
extensive disease preventing mastectomy at the time of recurrence. In one
series of 30 patients failing locally after conservative surgery and
radiotherapy who underwent salvage mastectomy, no distant recurrences
were seen later than six years after initial local failure, and the overall
disease-free survival following salvage mastectomy was 58% at five years
and 50% at 10 years. [ref: 3,4,5]

All patients with recurrent breast cancer should be considered candidates for one of the ongoing clinical trials testing newly developed chemotherapeutic agents and biologicals in phase II clinical trials.

Treatment options:

Standard:

1. If visceral disease is absent, estrogen and progesterone receptor status is positive or unknown, and the disease-free interval exceeds two years:
   tamoxifen or oophorectomy for premenopausal patients, or radiation castration, if surgery cannot be performed [ref: 6]
   antiestrogen therapy with tamoxifen for postmenopausal patients
   estrogen therapy for postmenopausal patients
   progesterone therapy for postmenopausal patients
2. If visceral disease is absent and recurrence is localized: surgery and/or radiotherapy [ref: 2]
3. Patients who respond to additive hormonal therapy and then relapse should be considered for other forms of hormonal therapy such as those previously unutilized therapies in (1) above or:
   androgen therapy for pre- and postmenopausal patients
   aminoglutethimide
   corticosteroids
   transphenoidal hypophysectomy
   This type of ablative procedure should only be performed by physicians who have extensive experience with this operation and the postoperative management of patients which is often complex.
4. If visceral disease is present and estrogen and progesterone receptor status is negative, or the disease-free interval is less than two years:
   CMF: cyclophosphamide + methotrexate + fluorouracil [ref: 7]
   CAF: cyclophosphamide + doxorubicin* + fluorouracil [ref: 8]
   CMFP: cyclophosphamide + methotrexate + fluorouracil + prednisone [ref: 7]
   CMFVP: cyclophosphamide + methotrexate + fluorouracil + vincristine + prednisone [ref: 8]
   L-PAM: melphalan, for frail, debilitated patients [ref: 9,10]
   CA: cyclophosphamide + doxorubicin* [ref: 11]

*The potential for doxorubicin-induced cardiotoxicity should be considered in the selection of chemotherapeutic regimens for an individual patient.

Investigational:

1. If visceral disease is absent, estrogen and progesterone receptor status positive or unknown, and the disease-free interval exceeds two years, investigational protocols evaluating the role of hormonal therapy such as administration of tamoxifen to premenopausal women should be considered. [ref: 6]

2. For patients with recurrences after an initial response to hormonal manipulation, investigational protocols evaluating combination chemotherapy with or without hormonal manipulation or investigational hormonal therapies should be considered.

3. If visceral disease is present, estrogen and progesterone receptor status is negative, or the disease-free interval is less than two years, investigational protocols evaluating combination chemotherapy, newly developed chemotherapeutic agents and biologicals should be considered.

References:

1. Perry MC, Kardinal CG, Korzun AH, et al.: Chemohormonal therapy in advanced carcinoma of the breast: Cancer and Leukemia Group B protocol 8081.
   Journal of Clinical Oncology 5(10): 1534–1545, 1987

2. Chen KK, Montague ED, Oswald MJ: Results of irradiation in the treatment of locoregional breast cancer recurrence.
   Cancer 56(6): 1269–1273, 1985

3. Aberizk WJ, Silver B, Henderson IC, et al.: The use of radiotherapy for treatment of isolated locoregional recurrence of breast carcinoma after mastectomy.
   Cancer 58(6): 1214–1218, 1986

4. Breast Diseases
   Harris JR, Hellman S, Henderson IC, et al., Eds.
   Philadelphia: J.B. Lippincott, 1987
      Specific sites and emergencies: local recurrence
      Recht A, Hayes DF
      pp 508–524

5. Harris JR, Recht A, Amalric R, et al.: Time course and prognosis of local recurrence following primary radiation therapy for early breast cancer.
   Journal of Clinical Oncology 2(1): 37–41, 1984

6. Ingle JN, Krook JE, Green SJ, et al.: Randomized trial of bilateral

oophorectomy versus tamoxifen in premenopausal women with metastatic breast cancer.
Journal of Clinical Oncology 4(2): 178–185, 1986

7. Tormey DC, Gelman R, Band PR, et al.: Comparison of induction chemotherapies for metastatic breast cancer: an Eastern Cooperative Oncology Group trial.
Cancer 50(7): 1235–1244, 1982

8. Smalley RV, Lefante J, Bartolucci A, et al.: A comparison of cyclophosphamide, Adriamycin, and 5-fluorouracil (CAF) and cyclophosphamide, methotrexate, 5-fluorouracil, vincristine and prednisone (CMFVP) in patients with advanced breast cancer: a Southeastern Cancer Study Group project.
Breast Cancer Research and Treatment 3(2): 209–220, 1983

9. Canellos GP, Pocock SJ, Taylor SG, et al.: Combination chemotherapy for metastatic breast carcinoma: prospective comparison of multiple drug therapy with L-phenylalanine mustard.
Cancer 38(5): 1882–1886, 1976

10. Carbone PP, Bauer M, Band PR, et al.: Chemotherapy of disseminated breast cancer: current status and prospects.
Cancer 39(Suppl 6): 2916–2922, 1977

11. Tranum BL, McDonald B, Thigpen T, et al.: Adriamycin combinations in advanced breast cancer: a Southwest Oncology Group study.
Cancer 49(5): 835–839, 1982

*Display complete. Press CR to return to previous menu.

CANCER INFORMATION MENU

Breast Cancer

Information for Patients   State-of-the-Art Information

	4 Prognosis
1 Prognostic Statement	5 Cellular Classification
2 Stage Explanations	6 Stage Information
3 General Treatment Options	7 Treatment by Cell Type/Stage

8 Display all information

9 Continuation options for citation abstracts, CANCERLIT searches and protocols

*Enter desired number and press CR.

> 9

CONTINUATION OPTIONS

BREAST CANCER

The following options are available for continuing your search. Your cancer diagnosis will be used automatically for all continuations.

1 Abstracts for literature citations in PDQ
2 CANCERLIT search statements
3 Investigational protocols
4 Standard therapy protocols

*Enter desired number and press CR.

> 1

CITATIONS BEING SORTED . . .

58 CITATION(S) REFERENCED.

REFERENCE
NUMBER
CITATION INFORMATION

1 Aberizk WJ, Silver B, Henderson IC, et al.: The use of radiotherapy for treatment of isolated locoregional recurrence of breast carcinoma after mastectomy. Cancer 58(6): 1214–1218, 1986

2 Adjuvant Therapy of Cancer IV Jones SE, Salmon SE, Eds. New York: Grune and Stratton, Inc., 1984 A summary of findings from NSABP: trials of adjuvant therapy Fisher B, Redmond C, Fisher ER, et al. pp 185–194

3 Advances in Breast and Endocrine Surgery Najarian JS, Delaney JP, Eds. Chicago: Year Book Medical Publishers, 1986 Breast reconstruction following mastectomy Cunningham BL pp 213–226

4 Bartlett K, Eremin O, Hutcheon A., et al.: Adjuvant tamoxifen in the management of operable breast cancer: The Scottish Trial. Lancet 2(8552): 171–175, 1987

*Enter desired number and press CR.

>

Reference
Number
Citation information

5 Baum M, Brinkley DM, Dossett JA, et al.: Controlled trial of tamoxifen as single adjuvant agent in management of early breast cancer: analysis at six years by Nolvadex Adjuvant Trial Organization. Lancet 1(8433): 836–840, 1985

6 Bonadonna G, Brusamolino E, Valagusso P, et al.: Combination chemotherapy as an adjuvant treatment in operable breast cancer. New England Journal of Medicine 294(8): 405–410, 1976

7 Breast Cancer—Diagnosis and Treatment Ariel IM, Cleary JB, Eds. New York: McGraw-Hill, 1987 Ch 16: The management of clinically nonpalpable breast cancer Leis HP, Cammarata A, LaRaja RD pp 205–223

8 Breast Diseases Harris JR, Hellman S, Henderson IC, et al., Eds. Philadelphia: J.B. Lippincott, 1987 Specific sites and emergencies: local recurrence Recht A, Hayes DF pp 508–524

*Enter desired number and press CR.

>

Reference
Number
Citation information

9 Buzdar AU, Blumenschein GR, Smith TL, et al.: Adjuvant chemotherapy with fluorouracil, doxorubicin, and cyclophosphamide, with or without bacillus Calmette-Guerin and with or without irradiation in operable breast cancer. Cancer 53(3): 384–389, 1984

10 Buzdar AU, Smith TL, Powell KC, et al.: Effect of timing of initiation
    of adjuvant chemotherapy on disease-free survival in breast cancer.
    Breast Cancer Research and Treatment 2(2): 163–169, 1982

11 Canellos GP, Pocock SJ, Taylor SG, et al.: Combination
    chemotherapy for metastatic breast carcinoma: prospective
    comparison of multiple drug therapy with L-phenylalanine mustard.
    Cancer 38(5): 1882–1886, 1976

12 Carbone PP, Bauer M, Band PR, et al.: Chemotherapy of
    disseminated breast cancer: current status and prospects. Cancer
    39(Suppl 6): 2916–2922, 1977

*Enter desired number and press CR.

>

Reference
Number
Citation information

13 Cascinelli N, Greco M, Bufalino R, et al.: Prognosis of breast cancer
    with axillary node metastases after surgical treatment only. European
    Journal of Cancer and Clinical Oncology 23(6): 795–799, 1987

14 Chen KK, Montague ED, Oswald MJ: Results of irradiation in the
    treatment of locoregional breast cancer recurrence. Cancer 56(6):
    1269–1273, 1985

15 Coulson PB, Thornthwaite JT, Woolley TW, et al.: Prognostic
    indicators including DNA histogram type, receptor content, and
    staging related to human breast cancer patient survival. Cancer
    Research 44(9): 4187–4196, 1984

16 Cummings FJ, Gray R, Davis TE, et al.: Adjuvant tamoxifen treatment
    of elderly women with stage II breast cancer: a double-blind
    comparison with placebo. Annals of Internal Medicine 103(3):
    324–329, 1985

*Enter desired number and press CR.

>

Reference
Number
Citation information

17 Davis BW, Gelber RD, Goldhirsch A, et al.: Prognostic significance of tumor grade in clinical trials of adjuvant therapy for breast cancer with axillary lymph node metastasis. Cancer 58(12): 2662–2670, 1986

18 Feller WF, Holt R, Spear S, et al.: Modified radical mastectomy with immediate breast reconstruction. American Surgeon 52(3): 129–133, 1986

19 Fisher B, Bauer M, Margolese R, et al.: Five-year results of a randomized clinical trial comparing total mastectomy and segmental mastectomy with or without radiation in the treatment of breast cancer. New England Journal of Medicine 312(12): 665–673, 1985

20 Fisher B, Brown A, Wolmark N, et al.: Prolonging tamoxifen therapy for primary breast cancer: findings from the National Surgical Adjuvant Breast and Bowel Project Clinical Trial. Annals of Internal Medicine 106(5): 649–654, 1987

*Enter desired number and press CR.

>

Reference
Number
Citation information

21 Fisher B, Fisher ER, Redmond C, et al.: Tumor nuclear grade, estrogen receptor, and progesterone receptor: their value alone or in combination as indicators of outcome following adjuvant therapy for breast cancer. Breast Cancer Research and Treatment 7(3): 147–160, 1986

22 Fisher B, Glass A, Redmond C., et al.: L-phenylalanine mustard (L-PAM) in the management of primary breast cancer: an update of earlier findings and a comparison with those utilizing L-PAM plus 5-fluorouracil (5-FU). Cancer 39(Suppl 6): 2883–2903, 1977

23 Fisher B, Redmond C, Brown A, et al.: Influence of tumor estrogen and progesterone receptor levels on the response to tamoxifen and chemotherapy in primary breast cancer. Journal of Clinical Oncology 1(4): 227–241, 1983

24 Fisher B, Redmond C, Brown A, et al.: Adjuvant chemotherapy with and without tamoxifen in the treatment of primary breast cancer: 5-year results from the National Surgical Adjuvant Breast and Bowel Project Trial. Journal of Clinical Oncology 4(4): 459–471, 1986

*Enter desired number and press CR.

>

Reference
Number
Citation information

25 Fisher B, Redmond C, Fisher ER, et al.: Ten-year results of a randomized clinical trial comparing radical mastectomy and total mastectomy with or without radiation. New England Journal of Medicine 312(11): 674–681, 1985
26 Fisher ER, Fisher B, Sass R, et al.: Pathologic findings from the National Surgical Adjuvant Breast Project (protocol no. 4): XI. Bilateral breast cancer. Cancer 54(12): 3002–3011, 1984
27 Fisher ER, Redmond C, Fisher B: Pathologic findings from the National Surgical Adjuvant Breast Project: VIII. Relationship of chemotherapeutic responsiveness to tumor differentiation. Cancer 51(2): 181–191, 1983
28 Glucksberg H, Rivkin SE, Rasmussen S, et al.: Combination chemotherapy (CMFVP) versus L-phenylalanine mustard (L-PAM) for operable breast cancer with positive axillary nodes: a Southwest Oncology Group study. Cancer 50(3): 423–434, 1982

*Enter desired number and press CR.

>

Reference
Number
Citation information

29 Harris JR, Recht A, Amalric R, et al.: Time course and prognosis of local recurrence following primary radiation therapy for early breast cancer. Journal of Clinical Oncology 2(1): 37–41, 1984
30 Hortobagyi GN, Blumenschein GR, Spanos W, et al.: Multimodal

treatment of locoregionally advanced breast cancer. Cancer 51(5): 763–768, 1983

31 Hryniuk W, Levine MN: Analysis of dose intensity for adjuvant chemotherapy trials in stage II breast cancer. Journal of Clinical Oncology 4(8): 1162–1170, 1986

32 Hryniuk WM, Levine MN, Levin L: Analysis of dose intensity for chemotherapy in early (stage II) and advanced breast cancer. National Cancer Institute Monographs 1: 87–94, 1986

*Enter desired number and press CR.

>

Reference
Number
Citation information

33 Hryniuk WM: Average relative dose intensity and the impact on design of clinical trails. Seminars in Oncology 14(1): 65–74, 1987

34 Hutter RV: The management of patients with lobular carcinoma in situ of the breast. Cancer 53(Suppl 3): 798–802, 1984

35 Ingle JN, Krook JE, Green SJ, et al.: Randomized trial of bilateral oophorectomy versus tamoxifen in premenopausal women with metastatic breast cancer. Journal of Clinical Oncology 4(2): 178–185, 1986

36 Jones SE, Salmon SE, Allen H, et al.: Adjuvant treatment of node-positive breast cancer with Adriamycin-cyclophosphamide with or without radiation therapy: interim results of an ongoing clinical trial. Recent Results in Cancer Research 80: 162–169, 1982

*Enter desired number and press CR.

>

Reference
Number
Citation information

37 Kurtz JM, Amalric R, DeLouche G, et al.: The second ten years: Long-term risks of breast conservation in early breast cancer.

International Journal of Radiation Oncology, Biology, Physics 13(9): 1327–1332, 1987

38 Levene MB, Harris JR, Hellman S: Treatment of carcinoma of the breast by radiation therapy. Cancer 39(6): 2840–2845, 1977

39 Manual for Staging of Cancer American Joint Committee on Cancer Philadelphia: JB Lippincott Company, 2nd ed., 1983 Part II: Staging of cancer at specific anatomic sites pp 23–243 Ch 21: Breast pp 127–133

40 Martin JK, van Heerden JA, Taylor WF, et al.: Is modified radical mastectomy really equivalent to radical mastectomy in treatment of carcinoma of the breast? Cancer 57(3): 510–518, 1986

*Enter desired number and press CR.

>

Reference
Number
Citation information

41 McGuire WL, Clark GM, Dressler LG, et al.: Role of steroid hormone receptors as prognostic factors in primary breast cancer. National Cancer Institute Monographs 1: 19–23, 1986

42 Meyer JS: Cell kinetics in selection and stratification of patients for adjuvant therapy of breast carcinoma. National Cancer Institute Monographs 1: 25–28, 1986

43 Moot SK, Peters GN, Cheek JH: Tumor hormone receptor status and recurrences in premenopausal node-negative breast carcinoma. Cancer 60(3): 382–385, 1987

44 National Institutes of Health Consensus Development Conference statement: adjuvant chemotherapy for breast cancer. Journal of the American Medical Association 254(24): 3461–3463, 1985

*Enter desired number and press CR.

>

APPENDIX 2

Reference
Number
Citation information

45 Perry MC, Kardinal CG, Korzun AH, et al.: Chemohormonal therapy
in advanced carcinoma of the breast: Cancer and Leukemia Group B
protocol 8081. Journal of Clinical Oncology 5(10): 1534–1545,
1987

46 Recht A, Danoff BS, Solin LJ, et al.: Intraductal carcinoma of the
breast: results of treatment with excisional biopsy and irradiation.
Journal of Clinical Oncology 3(10): 1339–1343, 1985

47 Review of mortality results in randomized trials in early breast cancer.
Lancet 2(8413): 1205, 1984

48 Romsdahl MM, Montague ED, Ames FC, et al.: Conservative surgery
and irradiation as treatment for early breast cancer. Archives of
Surgery 118(5): 521–526, 1983

*Enter desired number and press CR.

>

Reference
Number
Citation information

49 Silvestrini R, Daidone MG, Di Fronzo G, et al.: Prognostic implication
of labeling index versus estrogen receptors and tumor size in
node-negative breast cancer. Breast Cancer Research and Treatment
7(3): 161–169, 1986

50 Smalley RV, Lefante J, Bartolucci A, et al.: A comparison of
cyclophosphamide, Adriamycin, and 5-fluorouracil (CAF) and
cyclophosphamide, methotrexate, 5-fluorouracil, vincristine and
prednisone (CMFVP) in patients with advanced breast cancer: a
Southeastern Cancer Study Group project. Breast Cancer Research
and Treatment 3(2): 209–220, 1983

51 Swain SM, Sorace RA, Bagley CS, et al.: Neoadjuvant chemotherapy
in the combined modality approach of locally advanced
nonmetastatic breast cancer. Cancer Research 47(14): 3889–3894,
1987

52 Tancini G, Bonadonna G, Valagussa P, et al.: Adjuvant CMF in

breast cancer: comparative 5-year results of 12 versus 6 cycles.
Journal of Clinical Oncology 1(1): 2–10, 1983

*Enter desired number and press CR.

>

Reference
Number
Citation information

53 Tormey DC, Gelman R, Band PR, et al.: Comparison of induction
   chemotherapies for metastatic breast cancer: an Eastern Cooperative
   Oncology Group trial. Cancer 50(7): 1235–1244, 1982

54 Tranum BL, McDonald B, Thigpen T, et al.: Adriamycin combinations
   in advanced breast cancer: a Southwest Oncology Group study.
   Cancer 49(5): 835–839, 1982

55 Veronesi U, Banfi A, Del Vecchio M, et al.: Comparison of Halsted
   mastectomy with quadrantectomy, axillary dissection, and
   radiotherapy in early breast cancer: long-term results. European
   Journal of Cancer and Clinical Oncology 22(9): 1085–1089, 1986

56 Veronesi U, Saccozzi R, Del Vecchio M, et al.: Comparing radical
   mastectomy with quadrantectomy, axillary dissection, and
   radiotherapy in patients with small cancers of the breast. New
   England Journal of Medicine 305(1): 6–11, 1981

*Enter desired number and press CR.

>

Reference
Number
Citation information

57 Veronesi U, Zucali R, Luini A: Local control and survival in early
   breast cancer: the Milan trial. International Journal of Radiation
   Oncology, Biology, Physics 12(5): 717–720, 1986

58 Woods JE: Breast reconstruction: current state of the art. Mayo
   Clinic Proceedings 61(7): 579–585, 1986

---

*Enter desired number and press CR.

>

CONTINUATION OPTIONS

Breast Cancer

The following options are available for continuing your search. Your cancer diagnosis will be used automatically for all continuations.

1 Abstracts for literature citations in PDQ
2 CANCERLIT search statements
3 Investigational protocols
4 Standard therapy protocols

*Enter desired number and press CR.

>4

NOTHING FOUND FOR LAST SEARCH CRITERIA.
NO VALID SEARCH CRITERIA WERE SPECIFIED
*PRESS CR TO CONTINUE.
>3

PDQ STANDARD PROTOCOL RETRIEVAL

YOU MAY SELECT PROTOCOLS BY:

1 ID number
2 Cancer diagnosis
3 Word search in protocol title
4 Treatment modality
5 Drug name

*Enter desired number and press CR.

>2

DIAGNOSIS SELECTION

1 By body system/site
2 By histologic tissue/type
3 By childhood cancer

*Enter desired number OR type in a diagnosis and press CR.

> breast

Searching. . .

BREAST retrieved 1 diagnosis

No standard protocols found for BREAST CANCER
Standard protocols are not available for all diseases at this time.

PDQ STANDARD PROTOCOL RETRIEVAL

YOU MAY SELECT PROTOCOLS BY:

1 ID number
2 Cancer diagnosis
3 Word search in protocol title
4 Treatment modality
5 Drug name

*Enter desired number and press CR.

> back

PROTOCOL TYPES

1 Investigational Protocols
2 Standard Therapy Protocols

*Enter desired number and press CR ("Return" or "Enter" key).

> 1

PDQ INVESTIGATIONAL PROTOCOL RETRIEVAL

YOU MAY SELECT PROTOCOLS BY:

1 ID number
2 Cancer diagnosis
3 Word search in protocol title
4 Phase of protocol
5 Treatment modality
6 Drug name
7 State

*Enter desired number and press CR.

> 2; breast

Searching. . .

BREAST retrieved 1 diagnosis

PDQ INVESTIGATIONAL PROTOCOL RETRIEVAL

89 PROTOCOL(S) RETRIEVED
DIAGNOSIS = BREAST CANCER

YOU MAY NARROW SET OF PROTOCOLS BY:

1 ID number
2 Cancer diagnosis (use NARROW or BROADER to decrease/increase protocols)
3 Word search in protocol title
4 Phase of protocol
5 Treatment modality
6 Drug name
7 State—or you may
8 Erase existing selection criteria
9 Go to Print Option Menu (pause is OFF)

*Enter desired number and press CR.

> 9

PROTOCOL DISPLAY OPTIONS

1 BROWSE through protocol titles with option to select one or more protocols for display.
2 SHORT display all protocols in short format.
3 MEDium display all protocols in medium format.
4 NAMES display all protocols and investigators.
5 LONG display all protocols in long format.
6 MODS display all protocols long plus dosage modifications.
7 CUSTom display all protocols in custom format.
8 Change Pause Mode (currently OFF)
9 Return to protocol menu.

*Enter desired number and press CR.

> 2

89 PROTOCOL(S) BEING SORTED. . .

NCI-MB-82   NCI-T83-1248N   01/27/88
NCI-76-C-198
Orchiectomy with or without Subsequent Adrenalectomy for Metastatic
Cancer of the Male Breast and Adjuvant Chemotherapy for Stage II Male
Breast Cancer
   Marc E. Lippman
   Medical Breast Cancer Section, MB, COP, DCT
   National Cancer Institute
   National Institutes of Health
   Building 10, Room 12C205
   9000 Rockville Pike
   Bethesda, MD 20892
   301-496-4150
   Lead Organization
      Clinical Oncology Program
      Bethesda   MD

MSHMC-1609   NCI-V87-0248   01/27/88
Phase III Randomized Comparison of Hormonal Therapy with Leuprolide
Alone vs Leuprolide/Tamoxifen in Premenopausal Breast Cancer Patients
with Metastatic Disease (Last Modified 10/87)
   Allan Lipton
   Milton S. Hershey Medical Center

P.O. Box 850
500 University Drive
Hershey, PA 17033
717-531-8677
Lead Organization
  Milton S. Hershey Medical Center
  Hershey   PA

EST-3185   INT-0077   01/27/88
SWOG-8697
Phase III Randomized Comparison of CAF (CTX/ADR/5-FU) vs CAF
Alternating with TsAVbH (STEPA/ADR/VBL/FXM) for Induction Therapy
and CMF(P)TH (CTX/MTX/5-FU/PRED/TMX/FXM) vs No Therapy for
Maintenance in Patients with Hormone-Insensitive Metastatic or Recurrent
Breast Carcinoma (Last Modified 12/87)
  Kishan J. Pandya
  St. Mary's Hospital
  89 Genesee Street
  Rochester, NY 14611
  716-464-3591
  Lead Organization
    Eastern Cooperative Oncology Group
    Madison   WI

EST-8186   INT-0075   01/27/88
NCCTG-873201   SWOG-8692
Phase III Randomized Comparison of Surgical Oophorectomy vs Medical
Oophorectomy with ZDX in Premenopausal Patients with Metastatic
ER-Positive or PgR-Positive Carcinoma of the Breast (Last Modified 09/87)
  William S. Dalton
  University of Arizona Cancer Center
  Section of Hematology/Oncology
  1501 North Campbell Avenue
  Tucson, AZ 85724
  602-626-0111
  Lead Organization
    Southwest Oncology Group
    San Antonio   TX

CLB-8741   01/27/88
Phase III Randomized Comparison of MEG at the Standard Dose vs 5
Times vs 10 Times the Standard Dose in Patients with ER-Positive or
ER-Unknown Stage IV Carcinoma of the Breast

Joseph Aisner
University of Maryland Cancer Center
22 South Greene Street
Baltimore, MD 21201
301-328-2565
Lead Organization
    Cancer and Leukemia Group B
    Brookline   MA

NCI-V86-0143   WCCC-CO-8612   01/27/88
Phase III Randomized, Double-Blind, Placebo-Controlled Toxicity Study of
TMX in Postmenopausal Women with Early Stage Breast Cancer
    Richard R. Love
    Wisconsin Clinical Cancer Center
    Room K4-662
    600 Highland Avenue
    Madison, WI 53792
    608-263-8600, 608-263-7066
    Lead Organization
        Wisconsin Clinical Cancer Center
        Madison   WI

NCI-T86-0222D   NCOG-6G852   01/27/88
Phase III Randomized Comparison of Conventional Fractionated
Radiotherapy with vs without BUdR in Patients with Tumors Metastatic to
the Brain (Last Modified 11/87)
    Victor Alan Levin
    Brain Tumor Research Center
    University of California-San Francisco School of Medicine
    783 HSW
    San Francisco, CA 94143-0520
    415-476-3878
    Lead Organization
        Northern California Oncology Group
        Belmont   CA

MDA-DM-8612   NCI-V86-0106   01/27/88
Phase III Randomized Trial of Adjuvant Therapy with FAC (5-FU/ADR/CTX)
vs FAC plus MV (MTX/VBL) vs TMX in Patients with Resected Stage
II/III/IV Breast Cancer
    Aman U. Buzdar
    M.D. Anderson Hospital and Tumor Institute

Box 78
1515 Holcombe Boulevard
Houston, TX 77030
713-792-2121
Lead Organization
    M.D. Anderson Hospital and Tumor Institute
    Houston   TX

MAOP-1185   NCI-V86-0091   01/27/88
Phase III Randomized Study of the Efficacy and Toxicity of Three Delivery
Schedules of ADR in Patients with Metastatic Breast Cancer
    Jacob J. Lokich
    Medical Center of Boston
    125 Parker Hill Avenue
    Boston, MA 02120
    617-739-6605
    Lead Organization
       Mid-Atlantic Oncology Program
       Washington   DC

EST-2185   01/27/88
Phase III Randomized Evaluation of MEG Alone vs MEG Following
Pretreatment with Premarin in Patients with ER-Positive Metastatic
Carcinoma of the Breast (Last Modified 11/87)
    Charles D. Cobau
    Toledo Clinic, Inc.
    4235 Secor Road
    Toledo, OH 43623
    419-473-3561
    Lead Organization
       Eastern Cooperative Oncology Group
       Madison   WI

CAN-NCIC-MA4   NCI-V84-0074   01/27/88
Phase III Adjuvant Post-Surgical TMX vs TMX plus CMF (CTX/MTX/5-FU)
in ER and/or PR(+) Postmenopausal Breast Cancer Patients with
Histologically Involved Axillary Nodes (Last Modified 12/87)
    Kathleen I. Pritchard
    Toronto Bayview Regional Cancer Centre
    2075 Bayview Avenue
    Toronto, Ontario M4N 3M5
    Canada

416-488-5801
Lead Organization
  Clinical Trials Group
  Kingston   ON

NCI-V85-0176   UCSF-250803-01   01/27/88
Phase III Pilot Study of Peri-Operative Adjuvant Chemotherapy with
Sequential MTX and 5-FU with CF in Patients with Stage I/II Breast
Cancer
  Christopher C. Benz
  Cancer Research Institute
  The Medical Center at the University of California, San Francisco
  Room M 1282
  505 Parnassus Avenue
  San Francisco, CA 94143
  415-476-4149
  Lead Organization
    Cancer Research Institute
    San Francisco   CA

NCI-T86-0097N   NCI-86-C-46   01/27/88
Phase III Prospectively Randomized Study of Adoptive Immunotherapy with
High-Dose Recombinant IL-2 Administered Alone vs High-Dose
Recombinant IL-2 Administered in Conjunction with Systemic Administration
of LAK Cells in Patients with Advanced Cancer
  Steven A. Rosenberg
  Surgery Branch, COP, DCT
  National Cancer Institute
  National Institutes of Health
  Building 10, Room 2B 42
  9000 Rockville Pike
  Bethesda, MD 20892
  301-496-4164
  Lead Organization
    Clinical Oncology Program
    Bethesda   MD

RTOG-8419   01/27/88
Phase III Randomized Study of Interstitial Thermoradiotherapy vs Interstitial
Radiotherapy Alone for Metastatic, Recurrent, or Persistent Tumors
  Bahman Emami
  Mallinckrodt Institute of Radiology
  Professional Offices

Suite 5500
Division of Radiation Oncology
4939 Audubon Avenue
Saint Louis, MO 63110
314-362-7034, 314-362-8500
Lead Organization
   Radiation Therapy Oncology Group
   Philadelphia   PA

CLB-8793   MAOP-1285   01/27/88
NCOG-NSABP-B-17   NSABP-B-17
Phase III Randomized Study of Postoperative Radiotherapy Following
Segmental Mastectomy and Axillary Dissection in Patients with
Noninvasive Introductal Adenocarcinoma of the Breast (Last Modified
09/87)
   Bernard Fisher
   University of Pittsburgh School of Medicine
   Department of Surgery
   914 Scaife Hall
   3550 Terrace Street
   Pittsburgh, PA 15261
   412-648-9720
   Lead Organization
      National Surgical Adjuvant Project for Breast and Bowel Cancers
      Pittsburgh   PA

MDA-DM-8501   NCI-V85-0137   01/27/88
Phase III Preoperative Chemotherapy with VACP (VCR/ADR/CTX/PRED)
plus Surgery and Postoperative Radiotherapy and Chemotherapy with
VACP vs MFV (MTX/5-FU/VBL) for Stage III Breast Cancer
   Gabriel N. Hortobagyi
   M.D. Anderson Hospital and Tumor Institute
   1515 Holcombe Boulevard
   Houston, TX 77030
   713-792-2817
   Lead Organization
      M.D. Anderson Hospital and Tumor Institute
      Houston   TX

RTOG-8411   01/27/88
Phase III Randomized Comparison of Radiotherapy plus Hyperthermia vs
Radiotherapy Alone in the Treatment of Patients with Head and Neck

Carcinoma, Breast Cancer, or Soft Tissue Sarcoma Amenable to
Potentially Curable Radiotherapy (Last Modified 10/87)
  Ronald S. Scott
  Del Amo Diagnostic Center
  3531 Fashion Way
  Torrance, CA 90503
  213-214-2424
  Lead Organization
    Radiation Therapy Oncology Group
    Philadelphia   PA

POA-74185   01/27/88
Phase III Hormonal Therapy with TMX vs High-Dose MPA in Adult Patients
with Advanced Breast Cancer
  Hyman Bernard Muss
  Bowman Gray School of Medicine
  Section Hematology/Oncology
  300 South Hawthorne Road
  Winston-Salem, NC 27103
  919-748-4397
  Lead Organization
    Piedmont Oncology Association Regional Cooperative Group
    Winston-Salem   NC

POA-74285   01/27/88
Phase III Comparison of High- vs Low-Dose MEG in Patients with
Advanced Carcinoma of the Breast (Last Modified 12/87)
  Hyman Bernard Muss
  Bowman Gray School of Medicine
  Section Hematology/Oncology
  300 South Hawthorne Road
  Winston-Salem, NC 27103
  919-748-4397
  Lead Organization
    Piedmont Oncology Association Regional Cooperative Group
    Winston-Salem   NC

MAYO-853251   NCCTG-853251   01/27/88
Phase III Comparison of TMX/PRDL vs TMX/Placebo in Postmenopausal
Women with Advanced Carcinoma of the Breast (Last Modified 12/87)
  James N. Ingle
  Mayo Clinic

Division of Medical Oncology
200 First Street Southwest
Rochester, MN 55905
507-284-2511
Lead Organization
  North Central Cancer Treatment Group
  Rochester   MN

BRMP-8607   NCI-MB-198   01/27/88
NCI-T84-0518N   NCI-84-C-216B
NCI-86-C-188
Phase III Multimodality Approach to Patients with Inflammatory and
Locally Advanced Noninflammatory Stage III Carcinoma of the Breast and
Metastatic (Stage IV) Breast Carcinoma
  Marc E. Lippman
  Medical Breast Cancer Section, MB, COP, DCT
  National Cancer Institute
  National Institutes of Health
  Building 10, Room 12C205
  9000 Rockville Pike
  Bethesda, MD 20892
  301-496-4150
  Lead Organization
    Clinical Oncology Program
    Bethesda   MD

CLB-8541   01/27/88
Phase III Randomized Study of Adjuvant Chemotherapy with Intensive CDF
(CTX/ADR/5-FU) for Four Months vs Low-Dose CDF for Four Months vs
Standard-Dose CDF for Six Months in Patients with Node-Positive Stage II
Breast Cancer
  Daniel R. Budman
  North Shore University Hospital
  Division of Medical Oncology
  300 Community Drive
  Manhasset, NY 11030
  516-562-4160
  Lead Organization
    Cancer and Leukemia Group B
    Brookline   MA

MAOP-1684   NCOG-NSABP-B-16   01/27/88
NSABP-B-16
Phase III Randomized Comparison of Adjuvant Chemohormonal Therapy
with ACT (ADR/CTX/TMX) vs PAFT (L-PAM/ADR/5-FU/TMX) vs TMX
Alone in Patients Aged 50 Years and Older with Potentially Curable
Breast Carcinoma
   Bernard Fisher
   University of Pittsburgh School of Medicine
   Department of Surgery
   914 Scaife Hall
   3550 Terrace Street
   Pittsburgh, PA 15261
   412-648-9720
   Lead Organization
      National Surgical Adjuvant Project for Breast and Bowel Cancers
      Pittsburgh   PA

MAOP-1784   NCOG-NSABP-B-15   01/27/88
NSABP-B-15
Phase III Randomized Comparison of Adjuvant Chemotherapy with AC
(ADR/CTX) vs AC Plus Reinduction with Parenteral CMF (Intravenous
CTX/MTX/5-FU) vs Conventional CMF in Patients with Totally Resected
Breast Cancer with Positive Nodes
   Bernard Fisher
   University of Pittsburgh School of Medicine
   Department of Surgery
   914 Scaife Hall
   3550 Terrace Street
   Pittsburgh, PA 15261
   412-648-9720
   Lead Organization
      National Surgical Adjuvant Project for Breast and Bowel Cancers
      Pittsburgh   PA

NCI-T83-1038D   NYU-8305   01/27/88
Phase III Randomized Trial of Cardioprotection with ICRF-187 in Patients
with Advanced Breast Cancer Treated with FAC (5-FU/ADR/CTX)
   James L. Speyer
   New York University Medical Center
   Professional Building
   Department of Oncology, Suite 4J
   530 First Avenue

New York, NY 10016
212-340-7227
Lead Organization
  New York University Medical Center
  New York   NY

EST-5186   SWOG-8313   01/27/88
Phase III Adjuvant Chemotherapy with Short-Term Intensive FAC-M
(5-FU/ADR/CTX/MTX) vs CMFVP (CTX/MTX/5-FU/VCR/PRED) for
ER-Negative, Stage II/III Breast Carcinoma (Last Modified 12/87)
  Robert M. O'Bryan
  Henry Ford Hospital
  Division of Medical Oncology
  2799 West Grand Boulevard
  Detroit, MI 48202
  313-876-1852
  Lead Organization
    Southwest Oncology Group
    San Antonio   TX

SWOG-8312   01/27/88
Phase III Endocrine Therapy with MEG vs AGT/HC vs MEG plus
AGT/HC in Postmenopausal Women with Disseminated, TMX-Refractory
Breast Cancer
  James E. Congdon
  Everett Hematology-Oncology Association
  Suite 303
  4310 Colby Avenue
  Everett, WA 98203
  206-258-9388
  Lead Organization
    Southwest Oncology Group
    San Antonio   TX

MAOP-1184   01/27/88
Phase III Randomized Study of the Effect of MTX Dose and Interval
Between MTX and 5-FU in Patients with Recurrent and/or Disseminated
Breast Carcinoma Treated with CMF (CTX/MTX/5-FU)
  James D. Ahlgren
  Vincent T. Lombardi Cancer Research Center
  Georgetown University Medical Center
  Division of Medical Oncology

3800 Reservoir Road NW
Washington, DC 20007
202-625-7188
Lead Organization
  Mid-Atlantic Oncology Program
  Washington   DC

MI-BR-2   01/27/88
Phase III Adjuvant Study of Immunotherapy with BCG, Chemotherapy with
CMF (CTX/MTX/5-FU), and Radiotherapy, Alone and in Various
Combinations, in Patients with Breast Cancer Who Have Undergone
Mastectomy
  Robert L. Kerry
  St. Joseph's Mercy Hospital
  P.O. Box 995
  5301 East Huron River Drive
  Ann Arbor, MI 48106
  313-434-2800
  Lead Organization
    St. Joseph's Mercy Hospital
    Ann Arbor   MI

MI-BR-1   01/27/88
Phase III Chemotherapy with CMF (CTX/MTX/5-FU) and/or
Immunotherapy with BCG in Stage IV Disseminated Breast Cancer
  Robert L. Kerry
  St. Joseph's Mercy Hospital
  P.O. Box 995
  5301 East Huron River Drive
  Ann Arbor, MI 48106
  313-434-2800
  Lead Organization
    St. Joseph's Mercy Hospital
    Ann Arbor   MI

EST-4186   SWOG-7827   01/27/88
Phase III Randomized Trial of Various Adjuvant Therapies Using
Chemotherapy with CMFVP (CTX/MTX/5-FU/VCR/PRED) and/or
Hormonal Therapy with TMX or Oophorectomy for ER-Positive Stage II
Breast Cancer
  Saul E. Rivkin
  Tumor Institute of Swedish Hospital Medical Center

Arnold Medical Pavilion
1221 Madison Street
Seattle, WA 98104
206-386-2323
Lead Organization
    Southwest Oncology Group
    San Antonio   TX

SEG-BRE-83307R-T   01/27/88
Phase III Randomized Comparison of Adjuvant Combination
Chemotherapy with CAF (CTX/ADR/5-FU) vs CMF (CTX/MTX/5-FU) at
Maximal Tolerated Doses Following Mastectomy or Tylectomy for Breast
Cancer with Positive Axillary Nodes (Last Modified 12/87)
    John Topham Carpenter, Jr.
    The University of Alabama at Birmingham
    Division of Hematology-Oncology
    University Station
    Birmingham, AL 35294
    205-934-2084
    Lead Organization
        Southeastern Cancer Study Group
        Birmingham   AL

RTOG-8306   01/27/88
Phase III Radiotherapy with Boost of Electrons vs Interstitial Implant for
Nonmetastatic Adenocarcinoma of the Breast (Last Modified 10/87)
    Barbara Fowble
    Hospital of the University of Pennsylvania
    Department of Radiation Therapy
    3400 Spruce Street
    Philadelphia, PA 19104
    215-662-3075
    Lead Organization
        Radiation Therapy Oncology Group
        Philadelphia   PA

RTOG-8206   01/27/88
Phase III Comparison of Local Field Irradiation with and without
Single-Dose Hemibody Irradiation for Control of Symptomatic Bony
Metastases (Last Modified 12/87)
    Colin A. Poulter
    University of Rochester Cancer Center

Box 647
601 Elmwood Avenue
Rochester, NY 14642
716-275-5625
Lead Organization
  Radiation Therapy Oncology Group
  Philadelphia   PA

MAOP-1584   NCOG-NSABP-B-14   01/27/88
NSABP-B-14
Phase III Double-Blind, Antiestrogen Therapy with Tamoxifen Following
Mastectomy for ER-Positive Breast Cancer with Uninvolved Axillary Nodes
  Bernard Fisher
  University of Pittsburgh School of Medicine
  Department of Surgery
  914 Scaife Hall
  3550 Terrace Street
  Pittsburgh, PA 15261
  412-648-9720
  Lead Organization
    National Surgical Adjuvant Project for Breast and Bowel Cancers
    Pittsburgh   PA

MAOP-1484   -   NCOG-NSABP-B-13   01/27/88
NSABP-B-13
Phase III Adjuvant Sequential Chemotherapy with MTX/5-FU for
ER-Negative Breast Cancer with Uninvolved Axillary Nodes
  Bernard Fisher
  University of Pittsburgh School of Medicine
  Department of Surgery
  914 Scaife Hall
  3550 Terrace Street
  Pittsburgh, PA 15261
  412-648-9720
  Lead Organization
    National Surgical Adjuvant Project for Breast and Bowel Cancers
    Pittsburgh   PA

MAYO-813252   NCCTG-813252   01/27/88
Phase III Randomized Comparison of CFP (CTX/5-FU/PRED) vs CMFP
(CTX/MTX/5-FU/PRED) for Locally Inoperable, Recurrent, or Metastatic
Carcinoma of the Breast

James N. Ingle
Mayo Clinic
Division of Medical Oncology
200 First Street Southwest
Rochester, MN 55905
507-284-2511
Lead Organization
    Mayo Clinic
    Rochester   MN

NCI-N83-6011   NCI-79-C-111B   01/27/88
Phase III Mastectomy and Axillary Dissection vs Excisional Biopsy, Axillary
Dissection and Definitive Radiotherapy with or without Chemotherapy for
Stage I/II Breast Carcinoma
    Judith L. Bader
    Radiation Oncology Branch, COP, DCT
    National Cancer Institute
    National Institutes of Health
    Building 10, Room B3B38
    9000 Rockville Pike
    Bethesda, MD 20892
    301-496-5457
    Lead Organization
        Clinical Oncology Program
        Bethesda   MD

NCI-MB-164   NCI-T83-1159N   01/27/88
NCI-82-C-129
Phase III Chemohormonal Therapy with CTX/MTX/5-FU/TMX for Patients
with No Evidence of Disease Following Resection or Radiotherapy for
Recurrent Breast Cancer
    Marc E. Lippman
    Medical Breast Cancer Section, MB, COP, DCT
    National Cancer Institute
    National Institutes of Health
    Building 10, Room 12C205
    9000 Rockville Pike
    Bethesda, MD 20892
    301-496-4150
    Lead Organization
        Clinical Oncology Program
        Bethesda   MD

CLB-8693   EST-1180   01/27/88
INT-0011   SWOG-8294
Phase III Adjuvant Chemotherapy with CMFP (CTX/MTX/5-FU/PRED) and
Evaluation of Biological Parameters in Node-Negative Operable Female
Breast Cancer
  Edward G. Mansour
  Cleveland Metropolitan General Hospital
  3395 Scranton Road
  Cleveland, OH 44109
  216-459-4394
  Lead Organization
    Eastern Cooperative Oncology Group
    Madison   WI

NCI-V87-0302   WVU-8502   01/27/88
Phase II Therapy with Naltrexone in Patients with Metastatic Breast
Cancer (Last Modified 12/87)
  Anthony J. Murgo
  West Virginia University Hospitals, Inc.
  Medical Center Drive
  Morgantown, WV 26506
  304-293-4229
  Lead Organization
    West Virginia University Hospitals, Inc.
    Morgantown   WV

FCCC-86808   NCI-V87-0283   01/27/88
Phase II Chemotherapy with M-VAC (MTX/VLB/ADR/CACP) in Patients
with Advanced, Measurable Breast Cancer (Last Modified 12/87)
  Beth L. Saren
  Fox Chase Cancer Center
  7701 Burholme Avenue
  Philadelphia, PA 19111
  215-728-2626
  Lead Organization
    Fox Chase Cancer Center
    Philadelphia   PA

CHNMC-IRB-7020   NCI-V87-0258   01/27/88
Phase II Chemotherapy with 5-FU/High-Dose FA as First- or Second-Line
Treatment in Patients with Advanced Breast Cancer (Last Modified 11/87)
  Kim Allyson Margolin
  City of Hope National Medical Center

Department of Medical Oncology and Therapeutics Research
1500 East Duarte Road
Duarte, CA 91010
818-359-8111
Lead Organization
  City of Hope National Medical Center
  Duarte   CA

CLB-8782   01/27/88
Phase II Pilot Study of Adjuvant CAF (CPA/ADR/5-FU) Followed by
High-Dose CPA/CDDP/BCNU and Autologous Bone Marrow Support in
Patients with Stage II Breast Cancer and Ten or More Positive Nodes
(Last Modified 10/87)
  William P. Peters
  Duke University Medical Center
  Box 3961
  Erwin Road
  Durham, NC 27710
  919-684-6707
  Lead Organization
    Cancer and Leukemia Group B
    Brookline   MA

BGSM-74187   NCI-V87-0208   01/27/88
Phase II Study of Fluoxymesterone in Patients with Breast Cancer Who
Have Failed Tamoxifen and a Progestin
  Hyman Bernard Muss
  Bowman Gray School of Medicine
  Section Hematology/Oncology
  300 South Hawthorne Road
  Winston-Salem, NC 27103
  919-748-4397
  Lead Organization
    Bowman Gray School of Medicine
    Winston-Salem   NC

MDA-DM-87039   NCI-T87-0108C   01/27/88
Phase II Chemotherapy with Didemnin B for Patients with Metastatic
Breast Cancer (Last Modified 11/87)
  Khaled W. Jabboury
  M.D. Anderson Hospital and Tumor Institute
  Division of Medicine
  1515 Holcombe Boulevard

Houston, TX 77030
713-792-2817
Lead Organization
   M.D. Anderson Hospital and Tumor Institute
   Houston   TX

MAYO-873251   NCCTG-873251   01/27/88

Phase II Combination Chemotherapy with Continuous Infusion
VP-16/CDDP in Women with Metastatic Breast Cancer
   James Edward Krook
   The Duluth Clinic, Ltd.
   400 East 3rd Street
   Duluth, MN 55805
   218-722-8364
   Lead Organization
      North Central Cancer Treatment Group
      Rochester   MN

CLB-8743   01/27/88

Phase II Pilot Study of Adjuvant Chemotherapy with Intensive VPCMF
(VCR/PRED/CPA/MTX/5-FU) plus (in Lumpectomy Patients) Radiotherapy
Followed by Intensive Chemotherapy with ADR in Patients with Stage II or
III Breast Cancer
   Sushil Bhardwaj
   Mount Sinai Medical Center
   One Gustave L. Levy Place
   New York, NY 10029
   212-650-6361
   Lead Organization
      Cancer and Leukemia Group B
      Brookline   MA

MDA-DM-8645   NCI-V87-0169   01/27/88

Phase II Randomized Study of Intra-Arterial vs Intravenous Combination
Chemotherapy with FAC (5-FU/ADR/CTX) in Patients with Breast Cancer
Metastatic to the Liver
   Giuseppe Fraschini
   Medical Breast Service
   M.D. Anderson Hospital and Tumor Institute
   6723 Bertner Avenue
   Houston, TX 77030
   713-792-2817

Lead Organization
    M.D. Anderson Hospital and Tumor Institute
    Houston   TX

MDA-DM-8634   NCI-V87-0170   01/27/88
Phase II Feasibility Study of Continuous Infusion 5-FU and Concomitant
Total Brain Irradiation in the Management of Brain Metastases in Patients
with Advanced Breast Cancer
    Khaled W. Jabboury
    M.D. Anderson Hospital and Tumor Institute
    Division of Medicine
    1515 Holcombe Boulevard
    Houston, TX 77030
    713-792-2817
    Lead Organization
        M.D. Anderson Hospital and Tumor Institute
        Houston   TX

MAYO-863001   NCCTG-863001   01/27/88
Phase II Pilot Study of Chemotherapy with ADR Alternating with CMF
(CTX/MTX/5-FU) plus Surgery and/or Radiotherapy in Patients with
Local-Regionally Advanced Breast Cancer
    Charles L. Loprinzi
    Mayo Clinic
    200 First Street Southwest
    Rochester, MN 55905
    507-284-2511
    Lead Organization
        North Central Cancer Treatment Group
        Rochester   MN

MAYO-863201   NCI-T86-0234C   01/27/88
Phase II Study of Chemotherapy with 5-FU plus Leucovorin in Women with
Advanced Breast Cancer (Last Modified 11/87)
    Charles L. Loprinzi
    Mayo Clinic
    200 First Street Southwest
    Rochester, MN 55905
    507-284-2511
    Lead Organization
        Mayo Clinic
        Rochester   MN

MRH-860306 NCI-V86-0047 01/27/88
Phase II Pilot Study of Late Intensification Therapy with CTX/Thiotepa plus
Autologous BMT Following Induction with LOMAC
(CF/VCR/MTX/ADR/CTX) in Patients with Stage IV Breast Cancer
   Jacob D. Bitran
   Michael Reese Hospital and Medical Center
   Division of Oncology
   Lake Shore Drive at 31st Street
   Chicago, IL 60616
   312-791-5559, 312-791-5557
   Lead Organization
      Michael Reese Hospital and Medical Center
      Chicago   IL

MDA-DM-8632 NCI-V86-0105 01/27/88
Phase II Chemotherapy with ARA-C in Patients with Leptomeningeal
Metastases from Breast Cancer
   Frankie Ann Holmes
   Medical Breast Service
   M.D. Anderson Hospital and Tumor Institute
   Box 78
   6723 Bertner Avenue
   Houston, TX 77030
   713-792-2817
   Lead Organization
      M.D. Anderson Hospital and Tumor Institute
      Houston   TX

EST-PA-185 01/27/88
Phase II Pilot Study of Chemotherapy with CDDP/5-FU in Patients with
Recurrent Metastatic Breast Adenocarcinoma
   Omer Kucuk
   Veterans Administration Medical Center
   Building 50, Room 129
   North Chicago, IL 60064
   312-578-3342
   Lead Organization
      Eastern Cooperative Oncology Group
      Madison   WI

NCI-T86-0181D   YALE-HIC-3909   01/27/88
Phase II Evaluation of Trifluoperazine to Overcome Doxorubicin Resistance
in Patients with Breast Cancer
   William N. Hait
   Yale University School of Medicine
   333 Cedar Street
   New Haven, CT 06510
   203-785-4175
   Lead Organization
      Yale University School of Medicine
      New Haven   CT

CLB-8642   01/27/88
Phase III Master Protocol for Randomized Comparison of Single-agent
Chemotherapy vs Standard Therapy with CAF (CTX/ADR/5-FU) in
Previously Untreated Patients with Stage IV Breast Carcinoma—L-PAM
and Other Phase II Agents (Last Modified 11/87)
   Mary E. Costanza
   University of Massachusetts Medical Center
   Department of Medicine
   55 Lake Avenue North
   Worcester, MA 01605
   617-856-3902
   Lead Organization
      Cancer and Leukemia Group B
      Brookline   MA

MSKCC-8633   NCI-T86-0139D   01/27/88
Phase II Study of Palliative Radiotherapy plus Radiosensitization with
FAMP Using Two Administration Schedules in Patients with Multiple
Superficial Lesions from Melanoma, Soft Tissue Sarcomas, or Breast
Cancer
   Jae Ho Kim
   Memorial Sloan-Kettering Cancer Center
   Department of Radiation Oncology, Room 101 R
   1275 York Avenue
   New York, NY 10021
   212-794-6823
   Lead Organization
      Memorial Sloan-Kettering Cancer Center
      New York   NY

MDA-DM-8656   NCI-T86-0155C   01/27/88
Phase II Chemotherapy with Gallium Nitrate Administered by Continuous
Infusion in Patients with Refractory Metastatic Breast Cancer
   Khaled W. Jabboury
   M.D. Anderson Hospital and Tumor Institute
   Division of Medicine
   1515 Holcombe Boulevard
   Houston, TX 77030
   713-792-2817
   Lead Organization
     M.D. Anderson Hospital and Tumor Institute
     Houston   TX

EST-2186   01/27/88
Phase II Randomized Study of Continuous Infusion Chemotherapy with
ADR or 5-FU in Patients with Metastatic Breast Cancer (Last Modified
12/87)
   Alan K. Hatfield
   Carle Cancer Center Community Clinical Oncology Program
   Division of Hematology/Oncology
   Carle Clinic Association
   602 West University Avenue
   Urbana, IL 61801
   217-337-3010
   Lead Organization
     Eastern Cooperative Oncology Group
     Madison   WI

NCI-T86-0049D   YALE-HIC-3753   01/27/88
Phase II Chemotherapy with MF (MTX/5-FU) plus High-Dose Leucovorin in
Patients with Refractory Metastatic Breast Cancer
   Carol S. Portlock
   Yale University Comprehensive Cancer Center
   Section of Medical Oncology
   333 Cedar Street
   New Haven, CT 06510
   203-785-4110
   Lead Organization
     Yale University School of Medicine
     New Haven   CT

AECM-869   CHNMC-COH-6217   01/27/88
IDB-LAK-BREAST   LOY-7/86-6A
NCI-T86-01650   NEMCH-CSU-403
SWOG-8618   UCSF-804810-01
UTHSC-8565011283

Phase II Immunotherapy with High-Dose Recombinant IL-2 and Autologous LAK Cells in Patients with Metastatic or Unresectable Breast Cancer (Last Modified 12/87)
  Mario Sznol
  Investigational Drug Branch, CTEP, DCT
  National Cancer Institute
  National Institutes of Health
  7910 Woodmont Avenue
  Bethesda, MD 20892
  301-496-8798
  Lead Organization
    Investigational Drug Branch
    Bethesda   MD

SWOG-8571   01/27/88

Phase II Pilot Study of Induction Chemotherapy with FUVA (5-FU/VBL/ADR) Followed by Intensification with CTX, with Radiotherapy in Complete Responders, in Patients with Poor Prognosis Disseminated Breast Cancer
  Robert B. Livingston
  University Hospital
  RC-08
  1959 Northeast Pacific Street
  Seattle, WA 98195
  206-548-4125, 206-548-4100
  Lead Organization
    Southwest Oncology Group
    San Antonio   TX

IOWA-8501002   NCI-V85-0231   01/27/88

Phase II Chemotherapy with Lonidomine in Patients with an Advanced Refractory Melanoma or Breast Cancer (Last Modified 11/87)
  Gerald H. Clamon
  University of Iowa Hospitals and Clinics
  Department of Internal Medicine
  650 Newton Road
  Iowa City, IA 52242

319-356-1932
Lead Organization
  University of Iowa Hospitals and Clinics
  Iowa City   IA

ICC-86B1   NCI-T86-0076D   01/27/88
Phase II Master Protocol for the Study of New Agents in the Treatment
of Metastatic Adenocarcinoma of the Breast—DHAC
  Lary Jon Kilton
  640 Elm Road
  Barrington, IL 60010
  312-381-0834
  Lead Organization
    Illinois Cancer Council
    Chicago   IL

SWOG-8568   01/27/88
Phase II Combined Modality Therapy with Hormonal Therapy Using
Estradiol, Chemotherapy with FUVAC (5-FU/VBL/ADR/CTX) or FAC
(5-FU/ADR/CTX), Radiotherapy, and Surgery in Patients with Advanced
Stage III Breast Cancer
  Carol J. Fabian
  University of Kansas Cancer Center
  Division of Medical Oncology
  412 South Rainbow Boulevard
  Kansas City, KS 66103
  913-588-6029
  Lead Organization
    Southwest Oncology Group
    San Antonio   TX

NCK-MB-203   NCI-T86-0013N   01/27/88
NCI-85-C-198
Phase II Endocrine Therapy Using the LHRH Analog Leuprolide Acetate in
Combination with TMX/AGT/HC in Metastatic Breast Cancer
  Marc E. Lippman
  Medical Breast Cancer Section, MB, COP, DCT
  National Cancer Institute
  National Institutes of Health
  Building 10, Room 12C205
  9000 Rockville Pike
  Bethesda, MD 20892
  301-496-4150

Lead Organization
  Clinical Oncology Program
  Bethesda   MD

NCI-B85-0004C   OSP-83221   01/27/88
Phase II Study of the Effect of Intralesionally Administered Interferons on
the Size and Histology of Metastatic Tumor Nodules
  John J. Costanzi
  University of Texas Medical Branch Cancer Center
  Microbiology Building, Room G104, Rt J20
  Eleventh and Mechanic Streets
  Galveston, TX 77550
  409-761-1862
  Lead Organization
    University of Texas Medical Branch Hospitals
    Galveston   TX

DFCI-79049   NCI-T84-0176D   01/27/88
Phase II/III Pilot Study of Endocrine Therapy with Tamoxifen vs Tamoxifen
plus Aminoglutethimide in Premenopausal Patients with Metastatic Breast
Cancer
  I. Craig Henderson
  Dana-Farber Cancer Institute
  44 Binney Street
  Boston, MA 02115
  617-732-3472
  Lead Organization
    Dana-Farber Cancer Institute
    Boston   MA

JHOC-85041701   NCI-T85-0021D   01/27/88
Phase II Chemotherapy with Menogaril in Patients with Advanced Breast
Cancer
  Martin D. Abeloff
  Johns Hopkins Oncology Center
  First Floor, Room 128
  600 North Wolfe Street
  Baltimore, MD 21205
  301-955-8838
  Lead Organization
    Johns Hopkins Oncology Center
    Baltimore   MD

NCI-V85-0052   RPMI-PPC-679   01/27/88
Phase II Randomized Comparison of Combination Chemotherapy with CFP
(CTX/5-FU/PRED) vs CFPMV (CTX/5-FU/PRED/MTX/VCR) vs CA
(CTX/ADR) Administered Sequentially as First-, Second-, or Third-Line
Therapy in Patients with Metastatic Breast Cancer
   Dutzu Rosner
   Roswell Park Memorial Institute
   666 Elm Street
   Buffalo, NY 14263
   716-845-5947
   Lead Organization
      Roswell Park Memorial Institute
      Buffalo   NY

MDA-DM-8473   NCI-T84-0500C   01/27/88
Phase II Chemotherapy with High-Dose Mitoxantrone in Adults with
Advanced Breast Cancer (Last Modified 12/87)
   Frankie Ann Holmes
   Medical Breast Service
   M.D. Anderson Hospital and Tumor Institute
   Box 78
   6723 Bertner Avenue
   Houston, TX 77030
   713-792-2817
   Lead Organization
      M.D. Anderson Hospital and Tumor Institute
      Houston   TX

NCI-MB-186   NCI-T84-0322N   01/27/88
NCI-84-C-70
Phase II Prospectively Randomized Trial to Evaluate the Efficacy of a New
In-Vitro Drug Sensitivity Assay in Selecting Therapy for Patients with
Advanced, Previously Treated Breast Cancer
   Marc E. Lippman
   Medical Breast Cancer Section, MB, COP, DCT
   National Cancer Institute
   National Institutes of Health
   Building 10, Room 12C205
   9000 Rockville Pike
   Bethesda, MD 20892
   301-496-4150

Lead Organization
  Clinical Oncology Program
  Bethesda   MD

POA-74184   01/27/88
Phase II Randomized Comparison of Maintenance Therapy with CMFP
(CTX/MTX/5-FU/PRED) vs No Maintenance Therapy After Induction with
CAF (CTX/ADR/5-FU) in Previously Untreated Patients with Breast Cancer
  Hyman Bernard Muss
  Bowman Gray School of Medicine
  Section Hematology/Oncology
  300 South Hawthorne Road
  Winston-Salem, NC 27103
  919-748-4397
  Lead Organization
    Piedmont Oncology Association Regional Cooperative Group
    Winston-Salem   NC

NCI-T83-1033D   WCCC-CO-8214   01/27/88
Phase II Intensive Chemohormonotherapy as Primary Induction Followed
by Intensive Consolidation Radiotherapy in Patients with Metastatic
and/or Recurrent Breast Carcinoma
  Douglass C. Tormey
  Wisconsin Clinical Cancer Center
  Room K4/632
  600 Highland Avenue
  Madison, WI 53792
  608-263-8600
  Lead Organization
    Wisconsin Clinical Cancer Center
    Madison   WI

NCI-D81-048-515   WCCC-CO-8111   01/27/88
Phase II/III Multimodality Therapy with Surgery,
DBD/ADR/VCR/PRED/TMX/FLU/HMM/MTX/CF or
CTX/ADR/5-FU/TMX/FLU, plus Radiotherapy for Stage III Breast
Carcinoma
  William H. Wolberg
  Wisconsin Clinical Cancer Center
  Room K4-662
  600 Highland Avenue
  Madison, WI 53792

608-263-8604
Lead Organization
  Wisconsin Clinical Cancer Center
  Madison   WI

NCI-V87-0266   UTHSC-MS-85110   01/27/88
Phase I/II Trial of Systemic Hyperthermia plus CDDP Chemotherapy in
Patients with Advanced Malignant Melanoma and Other Neoplasms (Last
Modified 12/87)
  Joan M.C. Bull
  University of Texas Medical School
  Division of Hematology/Oncology
  Room 5016
  6431 Fannin Street
  Houston, TX 77030
  713-792-5450
  Lead Organization
    University of Texas Health Science Center
    Houston   TX

EST-PA-987   01/27/88
Phase I Combination Chemotherapy with High-Dose VP-16/L-PAM plus
Autologous Bone Marrow Rescue in Adults with Refractory Malignancies
  Hillard M. Lazarus
  University Hospitals of Cleveland
  Department of Medicine
  Division of Hematology/Oncology
  2074 Abington Road
  Cleveland, OH 44106
  216-844-3629
  Lead Organization
    Eastern Cooperative Oncology Group
    Madison   WI

IOWA-V87-0178   NCI-V87-0178   01/27/88
Phase I Chemotherapy with Oral 13-cis-Retinoic Acid on an
Every-12-Hour Schedule in Patients with Metastatic Malignancies
  Gerald H. Clamon
  University of Iowa Hospitals and Clinics
  Department of Internal Medicine
  650 Newton Road
  Iowa City, IA 52242

319-356-1932
Lead Organization
  University of Iowa Hospitals and Clinics
  Iowa City   IA

NCI-V86-0148   WCCC-CO-8697   01/27/88
Phase I Chemotherapy with Oral CTX, Bolus Intravenous ADR, and
Continuous Infusion 5-FU in Patients with Metastatic or Recurrent
Adenocarcinomas
  Guillermo Ramirez
  Wisconsin Clinical Cancer Center
  Room K4-628
  600 Highland Avenue
  Madison, WI 53792
  608-263-8600
  Lead Organization
    Wisconsin Clinical Cancer Center
    Madison   WI

DFCI-86125   NCI-T86-0297D   01/27/88
Phase I Chemotherapy with High-Dose CPA/TSPA/CBDCA Followed by
Autologous Bone Marrow Reinfusion in Patients with Advanced
Malignancies (Last Modified 10/87)
  Joseph P. Eder
  Dana-Farber Cancer Institute
  44 Binney Street
  Boston, MA 02115
  617-732-3767
  Lead Organization
    Dana-Farber Cancer Institute
    Boston   MA

DFCI-86014   NCI-T86-0026D   01/27/88
Phase I Study of High-dose IFX/CBDCA plus Mesna, Followed (if
Required) by Autologous Bone Marrow Rescue in Patients with Refractory,
Metastatic, or Locally Unresectable Malignancy
  Karen Antman
  Dana-Farber Cancer Institute
  Room F-271
  74 Binney Street
  Boston, MA 02115
  617-732-7339

Lead Organization
    Dana-Farber Cancer Institute
    Boston   MA

SWOG-8608   01/27/88
Phase I/II Chemotherapy with CDDP/DHAD in Patients with Advanced
Breast Cancer (Last Modified 12/87)
    John B. Craig
    Audie L. Murphy Memorial Veterans Hospital
    Division of Oncology, 111-J
    7400 Merton Minter Boulevard
    San Antonio, TX 78284
    512-694-4542
    Lead Organization
        Southwest Oncology Group
        San Antonio   TX

RTOG-8605   01/27/88
Phase I Radiosensitization with Continuous Infusion SR-2508 in Patients
Undergoing Interstitial or Intracavitary Radiotherapy for Solid Tumor
Control (Last Modified 10/87)
    C. Norman Coleman
    Joint Center for Radiation Therapy
    50 Binney Street
    Boston, MA 02115
    617-732-1889
    Lead Organization
        Radiation Therapy Oncology Group
        Philadelphia   PA

DFCI-84108   NCI-T85-0134W   01/27/88
Phase I Study of CBDCA with Autologous Bone Marrow Transplantation
in Patients with Advanced Malignancies
    Thomas C. Shea
    Dana-Farber Cancer Institute
    J.F. Building, Room 512
    44 Binney Street
    Boston, MA 02115
    617-732-3108
    Lead Organization
        Dana-Farber Cancer Institute
        Boston   MA

DUMC-336846R1   NCI-V85-0020   01/27/88
Phase I Combination Chemotherapy with High-Dose MTX/CACP plus CF
Rescue in Patients with Refractory Solid Tumors
  Andrew T. Huang
  Duke University Medical Center
  Department of Medicine, Box 3942
  Erwin Road
  Durham, NC 27710
  919-684-3127
  Lead Organization
    Duke University Medical Center
    Durham   NC

DUMC-7608611R2   NCI-T84-0505D   01/27/88
Phase I/II Combination Chemotherapy with High-Dose CTX/CACP/L-PAM
plus Autologous Bone Marrow Support in Patients with Metastatic Cancer
  William P. Peters
  Duke University Medical Center
  Box 3961
  Erwin Road
  Durham, NC 27710
  919-684-6707
  Lead Organization
    Duke University Medical Center
    Durham   NC

CTEPIS-0146   NCI-W83-0089   01/27/88
UTHSC-82305005
Phase I/II Mitoxantrone by Hepatic Arterial Infusion for Primary or
Metastatic Hepatic Tumor Refractory to All Known Therapy
  Geoffrey R. Weiss
  University of Texas Health Science Center
  7703 Floyd Curl Drive
  San Antonio, TX 78284-7845
  512-694-5186
  Lead Organization
    University of Texas Health Science Center
    San Antonio   TX

NCI-D83-048-628   WCCC-CO-8213   01/27/88
Phase I/II Adjuvant Therapy with
DBD/ADR/VCR/PRED/MTX/CF/FXM/TMX/HMM or CAFTH

(CTX/ADR/5-FU/TMX/FXM) Both with Radiotherapy for Resected Stage
I/II Breast Cancer (Last Modified 11/87)
   William H. Wolberg
   Wisconsin Clinical Cancer Center
   Room K4-662
   600 Highland Avenue
   Madison, WI 53792
   608-263-8604
   Lead Organization
     Wisconsin Clinical Cancer Center
     Madison   WI

*Display complete. Press CR to return to previous menu.

> EXIT

Goodbye NCI11

=== > > Please type END and hit CR to end PDQ session
< < === > END

QUERY SESSION TERMINATED
PDQ SESSION STARTED AT 13:54 AND ENDED AT 14:18 ON
01/27/88
YOU ARE BEING LOGGED OFF PDQ—IF YOU ARE AN ELHILL USER
AND WOULD LIKE TO LOG ON TO ELHILL, ENTER YES — — — > N
LOGGED OFF TSO AT 14:18:28 ON JANUARY 27, 1988
qe
NO CARRIER
IER

APPENDIX 3: AAMC—
Directory of American Medical Education

University of Alabama School of
Medicine
Birmingham, Alabama
(205)934-4011

University of South Alabama
College of Medicine
Mobile, Alabama
(205)460-7174

ARIZONA

University of Arizona College of
Medicine
Tucson, Arizona
(602)626-0111

ARKANSAS

University of Arkansas College of
Medicine
Little Rock, Arkansas
(501)661-5000

CALIFORNIA

University of California, Davis,
School of Medicine
Davis, California
(916)752-0331

University of California, Irvine,
School of Medicine
Irvine, California
(714)856-6119

University of California, Los
Angeles, UCLA School of
Medicine
Los Angeles, California
(213)825-6373

University of California, San
Diego, School of Medicine
La Jolla, California
(619)452-2230

University of California, San
Francisco, School of Medicine

San Francisco, California
(415)476-2342

Charles R. Drew, Postgraduate
School
Los Angeles, California
(213)463-4800

Loma Linda University School of
Medicine
Loma Linda, California
(714)824-4462

University of Southern California
School of Medicine
Los Angeles, California
(213)224-7001

Stanford University School of
Medicine
Stanford, California
(415)723-5019

COLORADO

University of Colorado Health
Sciences Center School of
Medicine
Denver, Colorado
(303)399-1211

CONNECTICUT

University of Connecticut School
of Medicine
Farmington, Connecticut
(203)674-2000

Yale University School of
Medicine
New Haven, Connecticut
(203)436-4771

DISTRICT OF COLUMBIA

George Washington University
School of Medicine and Health
Sciences
Washington, D.C.
(202)676-3266

Georgetown University School of
Medicine
Washington, D.C.
(202)625-7633

Howard University College of
Medicine
Washington, D.C.
(202)636-6270

FLORIDA

University of Florida College of
Medicine
Gainesville, Florida
(904)392-3701

University of Miami School of
Medicine
Miami, Florida
(305)547-6293

University of South Florida
College of Medicine
Tampa, Florida
(813)974-2196

GEORGIA

Emory University School of
Medicine
Atlanta, Georgia
(404)727-5650

Medical College of Georgia
School of Medicine
Augusta, Georgia
(404)828-0211

Mercer University School of
  Medicine
Macon, Georgia
(912)744-2600

Morehouse School of Medicine
Atlanta, Georgia
(404)752-1500

HAWAII

University of Hawaii John H.
  Burns School of Medicine
Honolulu, Hawaii
(808)948-8287

ILLINOIS

University of Chicago
Division of the Biological Sciences
Pritzker School of Medicine
Chicago, Illinois
(312)962-6500

University of Health
  Sciences/Chicago Medical
  School
North Chicago, Illinois
(312)578-3000

University of Illinois College of
  Medicine
Chicago, Illinois
(312)996-3500

Loyola University of Chicago
Stritch School of Medicine
Maywood, Illinois
(313)531-3000

Northwestern University Medical
  School
Chicago, Illinois
(313)908-8649

Rush Medical School of Rush
  University
Chicago, Illinois
(313)942-6913

Southern Illinois University
  School of Medicine
Springfield, Illinois
(217)782-3318

INDIANA

Indiana University School of
  Medicine
Indianapolis, Indiana
(317)274-8157

IOWA

University of Iowa College of
  Medicine
Iowa City, Iowa
(319)353-4843

KANSAS

University of Kansas Medical
  Center
Kansas City, Kansas
(913)588-5283

KENTUCKY

University of Kentucky College of
  Medicine
Lexington, Kentucky
(606)233-6582

University of Louisville School of
  Medicine
Louisville, Kentucky
(502)588-5184

LOUISIANA

Louisiana State University School
of Medicine in New Orleans
New Orleans, Louisiana
(504)568-4007

Louisiana State University School
of Medicine in Shreveport
Shreveport, Louisiana
(318)674-5000

Tulane University of Medicine
New Orleans, Louisiana
(504)588-5263

MARYLAND

Johns Hopkins University School
of Medicine
Baltimore, Maryland
(301)955-5000

University of Maryland School of
Medicine
Baltimore, Maryland
(301)528-7411

Uniformed Services University of
the Health Sciences
F. Edward Hebert School of
Medicine
Bethesda, Maryland
(301)295-3030

MASSACHUSETTS

Boston University School of
Medicine
Boston, Massachusetts
(617)638-8801

Harvard Medical School
Boston, Massachusetts
(617)732-1000

University of Massachusetts
Medical School
Worcester, Massachusetts
(617)856-0011

Tufts University School of
Medicine
Boston, Massachusetts
(617)956-6565

MICHIGAN

Michigan State University College
of Human Medicine
East Lansing, Michigan
(517)353-1730

University of Michigan Medical
School
Ann Arbor, Michigan
(313)763-9600

Wayne State University School of
Medicine
Detroit, Michigan
(313)577-1460

MINNESOTA

Mayo Medical School
Rochester, Minnesota
(507)284-3671

University of Minnesota
Duluth, Minnesota
(218)726-7571

University of Minnesota Medical
School–Minneapolis
Minneapolis, Minnesota
(612)624-1188

MISSISSIPPI

University of Mississippi School of
Medicine

Jackson, Mississippi
(601)984-1000

University of Missouri–Columbia
School of Medicine
Columbia, Missouri
(314)882-1566

University of Missouri–Kansas
City School of Medicine
Kansas City, Missouri
(816)276-1800

St. Louis University School of
Medicine
St. Louis, Missouri
(314)577-8000

Washington University School of
Medicine
St. Louis, Missouri
(314)362-5000

Creighton University School of
Medicine
Omaha, Nebraska
(402)280-2900

University of Nebraska College of
Medicine
Omaha, Nebraska
(402)559-4000

University of Nevada School of
Medicine
Reno, Nevada
(702)784-6001

Dartmouth Medical School
Hanover, New Hampshire
(603)646-7505

University of Medicine and
Dentistry of New Jersey
New Jersey Medical School
Newark, New Jersey
(201)456-4300

University of Medicine and
Dentistry of New Jersey
Robert Wood Johnson Medical
School
Piscataway, New Jersey
(201)463-1966

University of New Mexico School
of Medicine
Albuquerque, New Mexico
(505)277-2321

Albany Medical College of Union
University
Albany, New York
(518)445-5582

Albert Einstein College of
Medicine of Yeshiva University
Bronx, New York
(212)430-2000

Columbia University College of
Physicians and Surgeons
New York, New York
(212)305-3592

Cornell University Medical
  College
New York, New York
(212)472-5454

Mount Sinai School of Medicine
  of the City University of New
  York
New York, New York
(212)650-6500

New York Medical College
Valhalla, New York
(914)993-4000

New York University School of
  Medicine
New York, New York
(212)340-7300

University of Rochester School of
  Medicine and Dentistry
Rochester, New York
(716)275-3407

State University of New York
Brooklyn, New York
(718)270-1000

State University of New York at
  Buffalo
Buffalo, New York
(716)831-2775

State University of New York at
  Stony Brook
Stony Brook, New York
(516)444-2080

State University of New York
Health Science Center at Syracuse
Syracuse, New York
(315)473-5540

NORTH CAROLINA

Bowman Gray School of Medicine
  of Wake Forest University
Winston-Salem, North Carolina
(919)748-2011

Duke University School of
  Medicine
Durham, North Carolina
(919)684-3403

East Carolina University School
  of Medicine
Greenville, North Carolina
(919)757-2201

University of North Carolina at
  Chapel Hill School of Medicine
Chapel Hill, North Carolina
(919)966-4161

NORTH DAKOTA

University of North Dakota
  School of Medicine
Grand Forks, North Dakota
(701)777-2514

OHIO

Case Western Reserve University
  School of Medicine
Cleveland, Ohio
(216)368-2000

University of Cincinnati College
  of Medicine
Cincinnati, Ohio
(513)872-7391

Medical College of Ohio at
  Toledo
Toledo, Ohio
(419)381-4172

Northeastern Ohio University
College of Medicine
Rootstown, Ohio
(216)325-2511

Ohio State University College of
Medicine
Columbus, Ohio
(614)422-5674

Wright State University School of
Medicine
Dayton, Ohio
(513)873-3010

OKLAHOMA

University of Oklahoma College
of Medicine
Oklahoma City, Oklahoma
(405)271-4000

Oral Roberts University School of
Medicine
Tulsa, Oklahoma
(918)493-8033

OREGON

Oregon Health Sciences
University School of Medicine
Portland, Oregon
(503)225-8311

PENNSYLVANIA

Hahnemann University School of
Medicine
Philadelphia, Pennsylvania
(215)448-7000

Jefferson Medical College of
Thomas Jefferson University
Philadelphia, Pennsylvania
(215)928-6000

Medical College of Pennsylvania
Philadelphia, Pennsylvania
(215)842-6000

Pennsylvania State University
College of Medicine
Hershey, Pennsylvania
(717)531-8521

University of Pennsylvania School
of Medicine
Philadelphia, Pennsylvania
(215)662-4000

University of Pittsburgh School of
Medicine
Pittsburgh, Pennsylvania
(412)624-2489

Temple University School of
Medicine
Philadelphia, Pennsylvania
(215)221-3655

RHODE ISLAND

Brown University Program in
Medicine
Providence, Rhode Island
(401)863-3313

SOUTH CAROLINA

Medical University of South
Carolina College of Medicine
Charleston, South Carolina
(803)792-2081

University of South Carolina
School of Medicine
Columbia, South Carolina
(803)733-3210

University of South Dakota
School of Medicine
Sioux Falls, South Dakota
(605)339-6648

TENNESSEE

East Tennessee State University
Johnston City, Tennessee
(615)929-6315

Meharry Medical College School
of Medicine
Nashville, Tennessee
(615)327-6204

University of Tennessee College
of Medicine
Memphis, Tennessee
(901)528-5526

Vanderbilt University School of
Medicine
Nashville, Tennessee
(615)322-2145

TEXAS

Baylor College of Medicine
Houston, Texas
(713)799-4951

Texas A&M University College of
Medicine
College Station, Texas
(409)845-7743

Texas Tech University Health
Sciences Center School of
Medicine
Lubbock, Texas
(806)743-3000

University of Texas Health
Sciences Center at Dallas
Dallas, Texas
(214)688-3111

University of Texas Medical
School at Galveston
Galveston, Texas
(409)761-1011

University of Texas Medical
School at Houston
Houston, Texas
(713)792-2121

University of Texas Medical
School at San Antonio
San Antonio, Texas
(512)691-6451

UTAH

University of Utah School of
Medicine
Salt Lake City, Utah
(801)581-7201

VERMONT

University of Vermont College of
Medicine
Burlington, Vermont
(802)656-2150

VIRGINIA

East Virginia Medical School
Norfolk, Virginia
(804)446-5600

Virginia Commonwealth
University
Medical College of Virginia
School of Medicine
Richmond, Virginia
(804)786-9793

University of Virginia School of
Medicine
Charlottesville, Virginia
(804)924-0211

University of Washington School
of Medicine
Seattle, Washington
(206)543-1060

Marshall University School of
Medicine
Huntington, West Virginia
(304)526-0500

West Virginia University School
of Medicine
Morgantown, West Virginia
(304)293-4511

Medical College of Wisconsin
Milwaukee, Wisconsin
(414)257-8296

University of Wisconsin Medical
School
Madison, Wisconsin
(608)263-4900

INDEX

ABOUT THE AUTHOR

LAWRENCE C. HOROWITZ, M.D., is a physician who was director of the U.S. Senate Subcommittee on Health. He was also medical consultant to several of the largest corporations in America and is now a member of an investment advisory institution. He lives in San Francisco with his wife and four children.